Praise for *Weekend Wonder Detox*

"Michelle Schoffro Cook outlines six three-day programs designed to help readers look and feel better. Cook's plans combine detox recipes and nutritional advice with other healing therapies including mediation, acupressure and yoga."—*Inside Toronto*

Praise for *The 4-Week Ultimate Body Detox Plan*

"Michelle shares her compelling story of healing with wisdom and compassion as she gently guides you through this exceptional book. Read her book carefully and put into practice her simple, straightforward, commonsense principles, and you will be glad you did for the rest of your long and healthy life."—Harvey Diamond, #1 *New York Times* best-selling coauthor of *Fit for Life*

"Michelle's detox plan is an elegant, gentle, yet life-saving methodology, well-conceived through personal experience and thoroughly grounded in research. I heartily recommend it."—Meg Jordan, PhD, RN, editor-in-chief of *American Fitness*

"After the first week or so, you settle into a routine, get more adventurous in the kitchen, and start to really enjoy feeling good about the healthy choices being made. My *4-Week Ultimate Body Detox Plan* results: Lost—5 pounds; Gained—a much healthier attitude to food; Upside—My clothes fit better. I feel better. I'm eating better food and having way more fun in the kitchen. Insomnia is a thing of the past. Walking has become a regular part of my life. Downside—none."
—Robin Summerfield, contributing editor, *Calgary Herald*

the probiotic promise

Also by Michelle Schoffro Cook

*Weekend Wonder Detox: Quick Cleanses to Strengthen
    Your Body and Enhance Your Beauty*

60 Seconds to Slim: Balance Your Body Chemistry to Burn Fat Fast!

*The Ultimate pH Solution: Balance Your Body Chemistry
    to Prevent Disease and Lose Weight*

*The 4-Week Ultimate Body Detox Plan: A Program
    for Greater Energy, Health, and Vitality*

the
probiotic promise

Simple Steps to Heal Your Body from the Inside Out

• • • • • • • • • •

MICHELLE SCHOFFRO COOK, PhD, DNM, ROHP

Da Capo
LIFE
LONG

A MEMBER OF THE PERSEUS BOOKS GROUP

Designed by Jack Lenxo
Set in 11-point Sabon by the Perseus Books Group

Cataloging-in-Publication data for this book is available from the Library of Congress.

ISBN: 978-0-7382-1795-6 (hardcover)
ISBN: 978-0-7382-1796-3 (e-book)
First Da Capo Press edition 2015

Published by Da Capo Press
A Member of the Perseus Books Group
www.dacapopress.com

Note: The information in this book is true and complete to the best of our knowledge. This book is intended only as an informative guide for those wishing to know more about health issues. In no way is this book intended to replace, countermand, or conflict with the advice given to you by your own physician. The ultimate decision concerning care should be made between you and your doctor. We strongly recommend you follow his or her advice. Information in this book is general and is offered with no guarantees on the part of the authors or Da Capo Press. The authors and publisher disclaim all liability in connection with the use of this book.

Da Capo Press books are available at special discounts for bulk purchases in the U.S. by corporations, institutions, and other organizations. For more information, please con-tact the Special Markets Department at the Perseus Books Group, 2300 Chestnut Street, Suite 200, Philadelphia, PA, 19103, or call (800) 810-4145, ext. 5000, or e-mail special .markets@perseusbooks.com.

10 9 8 7 6 5 4 3 2 1

To Curtis, the love of my life and my soul mate.
I am blessed to share life with you and dedicate this
book to you. Never before have two loved more.

Contents

Chapter 1: The Health Secret We've All Been Waiting For 1

Chapter 2: The Surprising Worlds Within Your Body 15

Chapter 3: From the Common Cold to Superbugs: Probiotics to the Rescue 47

Chapter 4: New Hope for Serious Illnesses 79

Chapter 5: How to Select Probiotic Supplements 103

Chapter 6: Fall in Love with Fermented Foods 139

Chapter 7: Easy, Delicious, Probiotic-Rich Recipes 181

Metric Conversions 225

Appendix: The Cutting-Edge Research 229

Resources 241

Notes 247

About the Author 269

Acknowledgments 271

Index 273

Chapter 1

The Health Secret We've All Been Waiting For

"Health is a state of complete physical, mental and social well-being, and not merely the absence of disease or infirmity."

—World Health Organization

Anne Overcomes IBS

Anne, a stay-at-home mother with two young children, came into my office looking for a natural approach to what she suspected was *irritable bowel syndrome*. Test after test had ruled out colitis, Crohn's disease, colon cancer, and just about every other intestinal disease imaginable. She had read about irritable bowel syndrome and suffered from the symptoms of the condition, including abdominal cramping with alternating constipation and diarrhea, among others.

After reviewing the diet diary I had asked her to complete for the week prior to her appointment with me, I found she ate like most North Americans—a lot of junk. Because she was always chasing after a two-year-old (I'm sure most moms can attest that this is no small

Anne Overcomes IBS (continued)

task on its own!), trying to keep a clean home, balance her husband's hectic work and travel schedule with the needs of her mother who required ongoing care and attention, she often resorted to TV dinners or frozen packaged foods.

I explained to her that "you *really* are what you eat: what you eat is broken down into the building blocks of every cell, tissue, and organ in your body. So if you're suffering from ill health, that's a sign your body may be failing at the cellular level—not getting adequate nutrition to form healthy cells and tissues." I also discussed that our bodies are not meant to eat the myriad chemicals found in packaged foods, nor are they meant to ingest so much sugar. Although she insisted she didn't eat much sugar, I kept a couple of empty packages from frozen foods in my office and pointed out the number of grams of sugar each one contained. I also explained that we should never eat that much sugar at a single meal. Even if she didn't eat dessert, she had already eaten the equivalent in sugar at every meal whenever she ate these packaged foods.

She still didn't get what the "big deal" about sugar was. I explained that high amounts of sugar literally sent her body into crisis mode, causing her energy levels, moods, and bowels to respond. Depending on whether she was eating enough fiber on any particular day, that flood of sugar into her intestines might result in cramping, diarrhea, or constipation.

I asked her to eat a whole foods diet consisting of vegetables, a small amount of fruit eaten on an empty stomach, and lean protein and to gradually increase the amount of legumes, starting with only a tablespoon. I also encouraged her to avoid any food with more than ten grams of sugar at one time as well as any food with chemical ingredients she couldn't pronounce.

I also recommended a probiotic supplement that contained *Lactobacillus acidophilus* and *Bifidobacteria bifidum*, explaining that these probiotics were naturally present in her body when she was born and that the chemicals and sugar in her diet, among other lifestyle factors, had depleted her natural stores. I also conveyed that this product was completely natural and that I felt it was one of the best things she could do for irritable bowel syndrome.

A month later she came back, explaining that the constipation and diarrhea as well as the cramping were much better. She estimated that her symptoms had improved about 70 percent in only one month. Additionally, what surprised her the most was that she had so much more energy. Only a month ago she could barely keep up with her two-year-old but now was finding that she wanted to do more—go out more and spend more time in the park with her kids and even had more energy to make meals. A total convert to a healthier diet and probiotics, Anne now ensures her husband and children eat the same healthy diet.

Every time I open a health magazine or nutrition journal I see probiotics. Every time I turn on the television or browse through a health food store I observe claims for "probiotic-rich" foods and supplements, all claiming to offer hope in the treatment of illness and reversal of disease. Probiotics are being called the "supplement of the year" and "health food of the year" everywhere I turn. There is no doubt that the topic of probiotics is extremely popular right now.

Even if you are not involved in the health field like I am or have had little interest in health until now, you have probably still heard about probiotics in passing or seen the television commercials and magazine advertisements for the many foods, beverages, and supplements that contain or at least claim to contain probiotic cultures. You may enjoy your morning yogurt or afternoon yogurt snack with the hope of receiving the intestinal health benefits they offer. But even though you've probably heard about probiotics, you may still be wondering, *What exactly are they?* Scientists describe probiotics as "live microorganisms that, when administered in adequate amounts, confer a health benefit on the host."[1] Simply put, they are living bacteria and other microorganisms that have the ability to improve your health, boost your immune system, improve digestion, and increase your body's capacity to prevent or fight disease. Scientists around the world are making discoveries that are dramatically changing our collective medical history, holding the promise of significantly greater individual health and possibly even reversing many of the serious diseases that plague us in our modern age.

As a doctor of natural medicine and a health journalist for almost twenty-five years, I spend my days poring through the latest scientific research on foods, supplements, herbs, nutrients, oils, and natural therapies. In my earliest years of research I occasionally found studies on probiotics, but as the years progressed, so did the volume of research. Now hundreds of studies are being added to the collective literature on probiotics every year. We have probably doubled our total knowledge of probiotics in just the last couple of years. I worked with Anne, who I mentioned above, about twenty-three years ago. You'll recall that Anne complained of intestinal problems, namely, irritable bowel syndrome and abdominal cramping. At that time the only probiotic supplement options available included two strains of probiotics. When I recommended the product as part of her overall health-building program, she was reluctant to take them. After all, she conveyed, "*Lactobacillus acidophilus* sounds too complex to be natural," and Anne wanted a completely natural approach. I reassured her that not only was the product totally natural, they were intended to replenish bacteria that are naturally present in our bodies and in many food items. They worked remarkably for her. Jump ahead twenty-three years, and my clients actually come to my office asking for probiotics and concerned if there aren't many different strains. They want the most products with billions of live cultures and more strains than they can count. You'll find out later why this is not always the best idea. Nowadays it can actually be difficult to find a two-strain probiotic supplement like the one I used with Anne with great results. As the science advanced, so have the products. Now it's common for me to use probiotic supplements as my "go to" products for almost every client and condition. That's because they set the stage for the body's own innate healing.

What the Research Means for You

Not only did the volume of probiotic research skyrocket over the last couple of years, but scientists around the globe also began studying the effects of probiotics on diseases that go well beyond the gastrointestinal (GI) tract. They explored and are continuing to explore the effects of probiotics on everything from allergies and arthritis to depression and obesity. They even found probiotics that are effective against various types of cancer and HIV and AIDS. As if that weren't enough, probiotics are working when antibiotics and other medical interventions for serious infections fail. This research is shedding light on the role beneficial bacteria play in our health, and it goes far beyond our intestines. Study after study shows that probiotics are effective for healing and deserve a rightful place in our medicine cabinets, whether we are more comfortable with natural medicines or prefer pharmaceutical drugs.

That means that no matter where you fall on a spectrum of health to illness, you can experience the life-changing benefits probiotics offer. And if you're suffering from illness, you'll discover that *The Probiotic Promise*, which is the synthesis of all of the best research out there, offers promise and hope.

So much of this incredible research isn't even mainstream news; I wrote this book to share it with you with the hope that through *The Probiotic Promise* you will discover new ways to prevent illness, treat the health problems you're experiencing, transform your health, and experience the vitality that is your birthright. It incorporates the discoveries of some of the world's greatest scientists into an easy-to-follow approach that anyone can use to improve his or her health. This cutting-edge research offers the missing key to great health that can transform the body at the minutest level, restoring microbial balance that works through every system of the body, thereby restoring health in the process. Over time I believe that the collective research of these many great scientists all over the world will likely make our current "medical marvels" in the pharmaceutical world seem tiny in comparison to the power of probiotics.

Not Just for Gut Health

Exciting new research shows that some strains of probiotics are killing superbugs even when antibiotics stop working. Even better, research demonstrates that the superbugs do not develop resistance to probiotics in the way they learn to resist antibiotics! That's largely due to the complex structure of probiotics. By comparison antibiotics are quite simple in chemical structure. Superbugs can't outsmart probiotics the way they outsmart antibiotics, which is great news when you consider the rapidly growing accounts of antibiotic resistance: over 70 percent of all pathogenic bacteria in hospitals are at least minimally resistant to antibiotics.[2] You'll also learn in Chapter 3 how probiotics can assist in the treatment of infections. Probiotics are poised to become the weapon of choice against infections of the future.

Most people think probiotics, the bacteria found in yogurt, fermented foods, and supplements, are intended exclusively for digestive health. It's the myth that many authors, health professionals, and corporations perpetuate. And to be fair, it is likely because they probably aren't aware of the vast body of research that shows the benefits of probiotics beyond the GI tract. But that's just the tip of the iceberg of what these micro-miracle workers can do. Exciting new research reveals that healthy bacteria can heal a whole host of health conditions, including allergies, arthritis, celiac disease, depression, and brain disease, and can even help inhibit cancer, HIV, and AIDS. We'll discuss these conditions and the probiotics that help them in Chapter 4: New Hope for Serious Illnesses (except HIV and AIDs, which we'll discuss in Chapter 3).

Currently, people are needlessly suffering from many health conditions. That's because they're unaware of a critical piece of the healing puzzle: microbial balance within the body. Without addressing this foundation for health, their healing results may be short-lived or unsuccessful. By taking the right strains of *live* probiotic bacteria, in the right quantities and at the right time, a person's health can be transformed, increasing the body's resistance to future bouts with disease. Unfortunately, few people know what the right strains, quantities, or timing should be. Instead, most people take probiotics in an ad hoc manner and say they didn't work, but their lack of efficacy is a reflection of the misuse of probiotics. I'll explain more about how to choose and take probiotic supplements in Chapter 5: How to Select Probiotic Supplements, or how to propagate them in the food you make in your own kitchen in Chapter 6: Fall in Love with Fermented Foods.

Many corporations that manufacture yogurt, probiotic-containing beverages, and supplements aren't helping the situation

What's in It for You?

There are many benefits this book will offer you. You'll discover:

1. the rampant myths about probiotics—and how to avoid falling prey to them
2. why you should incorporate probiotics into your day-to-day life
3. the many research-proven health benefits of adding probiotics to your life, from digestion to infections, and so much more
4. why you'll want to make probiotics your "go to" natural remedy for a wide variety of concerns
5. how to select the best probiotic supplement for you at this time in your life
6. how your probiotic needs may change over your lifetime and vary greatly from one person to another
7. that many probiotic-rich foods go well beyond yogurt, that many yogurts aren't the health foods the companies claim, and that some are actually worse than doughnuts
8. how to add more probiotic-rich foods to your diet
9. how to make more probiotic-rich foods and why you'll want to, including delicious and nutritious probiotic-rich recipes to help you get started
10. a new and delicious way of eating that you'll want to continue for your lifetime

Ultimately, if you implement the suggestions throughout this book, you'll experience greater health, reduced likelihood of infections, and stronger immunity. If you're like most of my clients, you'll gain greater energy, vitality, and quality of life. Perhaps most importantly, you'll gain a greater respect and appreciation for your body and the probiotic helpers it relies upon.

either. Some companies claim that their products contain "live cultures" when they do not. Many claim their products contain "important prebiotics" when they are simply loaded with sugar, which can aggravate health conditions, like they did in Anne's case. And commercials with "dancing" abdominal cartoon-style molecules or fictitious names of bacteria ("BL Regularis," for example, which is a made-up name, albeit a trademarked one, and not a real type of probiotic bacteria) only further the confusion and misinformation. Those products that contain live bacterial cultures rarely contain the many cultures needed for strong disease resistance and often don't contain live cultures at all. You'll learn more about the many strains of beneficial bacteria in fermented foods in Chapter 6.

How to Use This Book

S ome of my earliest nutrition studies indicated that intestinal health was the key to vibrant health. Twenty-five years have passed, and now scientists have validated this belief with volumes of research. A tremendous opportunity awaits us as we incorporate a wide range of probiotics and probiotic-rich foods into our diet and lifestyle to prevent and, in some cases, even reverse disease. Even in those twenty-five years we've come a long way from believing that probiotics were essential for a healthy GI tract. It is true that probiotics are essential to a healthy gut, but they are also essential for a healthy brain, heart, immune system, and so much more. They are critical to our health, yet they are still the most overlooked part of a healthy lifestyle. I will share some of the most overlooked secrets of great health in this book.

I have spent the last quarter-century as a health journalist, author of sixteen books, and in earning advanced degrees in nutrition and health. During my research and writing I came across study after study of the benefits of various probiotic bacteria. Intrigued, I collected them in a file folder that eventually grew into a filing drawer full and, later, a cabinet full of the latest research on these health-promoting bacteria.

I've translated the medical jargon and the hundreds of scientific studies into real-life approaches you can use to improve your health immediately. I will share some of the most exciting research throughout *The Probiotic Promise*, but I have also included a separate appendix at the back of the book summarizing additional essential research, The Cutting-Edge Research, for those who want to delve deeper into the thought-provoking science behind *The Probiotic Promise*.

This research is transforming our understanding of our bodies, many health conditions, and even how to overcome these health concerns. I believe this research is so important that it is in the midst of revolutionizing our health care system from the current medical way of treating disease to a more natural, harmonious system of giving the body the tools it needs to overcome illness and restore health. That might seem like semantics, but it's not. Many drugs simply suppress symptoms but never restore health. Yet isn't health what we're all after? Remember that health is not just the absence of symptoms; it is the restoration of vitality, energy, and quality of life. And probiotics definitely play a role, as they are the foundational components of a healthy body.

The Probiotic Promise is the culmination of this startling research featuring the array of health benefits arising from these helpful flora. Although most people simply take the probiotic supplement their local health food store representative recommended to them, this one-size-fits-all approach to popping probiotic pills is really not that effective. There is no single strain of probiotic bacteria that is a magic pill for every health condition. The more effective way to get results with probiotic supplements is to find the scientifically proven strains of probiotics that are effective for the health condition(s) you face. The best probiotic for allergies is not the best probiotic for brain diseases, and the best ones for boosting immunity against cancer are not the best ones for depression, and so on.

Many people take an ad hoc approach to probiotics, expecting that the one-supplement-fits-all approach will miraculously cure them of whatever ails them. *The Probiotic Promise* will arm you so as to ensure that you are getting the best strains of beneficial bacteria for the specific health condition or conditions you are experiencing. You'll learn more about which strains of probiotics and probiotic-rich foods are best for your conditions in Chapters 4 to 6.

It will also guide you in your selection of high-quality probiotic supplements, explain how to tell whether the cultures in your yogurt are truly *live* (see the Yogurt Test in Chapter 5), and how to ensure they remain intact through the GI tract. It's important that you are empowered to take charge of your life. So I have presented vital healing information in a practical, do-it-yourself format that's easy to follow.

Supplements are only part of the equation; you can reap the benefits of probiotics by incorporating more fermented foods into your diet. I will also share the forgotten food-preservation techniques our ancestors used for hundreds, even thousands of years. Although these techniques were originally developed to preserve food, they also offer the health benefit of increased numbers of beneficial microbes of many different types. These probiotic-rich foods and beverages are also known as fermented or cultured foods. I will be using all three terms interchangeably throughout *The Probiotic Promise*. These foods are part of our forgotten heritage, and our ancestors ate them in large quantities, contributing to their ability to preserve food for use during winter when they couldn't grow fresh vegetables and in scarce times. These techniques are not archaic relics of a more primitive past; they turn good foods into healing superfoods that help prevent and reverse many kinds of diseases. You may be surprised to learn that fermenting these foods doesn't just boost their healing abilities; the fermentation process ramps up their nutritional value and makes otherwise boring and bland foods taste delicious. What's more, these nutritious and even life-saving cultured foods are simple to make at home and actually save time and make mealtimes easier, contrary to what you may have heard. Most of these foods require no special equipment.

Chapter 7 is devoted to recipes for some of my favorite delicious, naturally fermented, health-supportive foods. There are recipes that can be included in every meal, such as Savory Dairy-Free Greek-Style Yogurt, Curtis's Chocolate Banana Pro Smoothie, Soft and Creamy Dairy-Free Cheese, Fermented Green Tea (Kombucha), Green Chili Hot Sauce, Roasted Red Pepper Soft Cheese, Apple-Cabbage Kraut, Creamsicle Ice Cream, and many others.

Even if you have no interest in creating cultured foods, in this book you'll discover how readily available and affordable probiotics of many different varieties can help you overcome allergies, arthritis, cancer, diabetes, and other serious health conditions. Regardless your reason for reading *The Probiotic Promise*, I hope to share my passion for probiotic therapy, an approach to health that is almost unexplored and nothing less than miraculous.

And, as I mentioned earlier, this approach is about transforming health from the inside out as opposed to simply slapping a Band-Aid on a symptom or a condition. As an example, our medical approach of using antibiotics to rampantly kill bacteria in the body may work to kill an infection—although it may no longer work now that bacteria are becoming resistant, which I'll discuss in greater detail shortly. Probiotics, as the research shows, frequently work as well as and sometimes better than antibiotics when we already have an infectious disorder, but they are also an integral part of our bodies and their makeup, so restoring them helps to ensure our bodies function well, and we may avoid future infections altogether.

Probiotics vs. Antibiotics

You may be wondering how probiotics differ from antibiotics. Probiotics literally mean "supports life," whereas antibiotic means "against life." Within each of these words you'll actually find the method by which they work. Probiotics work in many different ways, but all of them support health so your body will be stronger to fight harmful pathogens. They primarily work by strengthening the beneficial bacteria in your intestines and elsewhere in your body. An increased number of beneficial microbes can also sway the "intermediate" microbes to act as beneficial microbes. Conversely, antibiotics indiscriminately kill microorganisms, both beneficial and harmful. With that rampant killing of microbes, harmful microbes can more readily settle and take hold in the body, leaving us vulnerable to infections. That's why so many people complain of getting a yeast infection or other type of infection or diarrhea and other uncomfortable symptoms after a period of antibiotic use.

Antibiotics may be beneficial in some instances and have saved many peoples' lives; however, it is the current overuse and misuse of them that is a serious problem. In this way they are playing a role in causing pathogenic bacteria to overgrow, causing infection, or, worse, to strengthen and cause superbugs. Moreover, the medical establishment's chosen weapon against superbugs—antibiotics—are becoming less and less effective against these infections. That's because the superbugs have adapted to the genetic composition of the antibiotics—in essence, they're outsmarting them!

As Dr. Hiromi Shinya so aptly stated, "We cannot find our way to health by trying to destroy whole categories of life."[3] Yet that is exactly the approach we have taken with antibiotics. We administer antibiotics whether we have a cold, flu, or some other infection even though antibiotics don't work on colds or flu, as they are viral illnesses, not bacterial ones. Even if the infection is bacterial, we indiscriminately kill beneficial bacteria that assist us in eliminating infections along with the infection-causing bacteria when we take antibiotics.

I'm not suggesting that we should eliminate antibiotics. As I mentioned, they have saved many people's lives; however, our current use is dangerous and causing the development of superbugs that pose a serious threat to our health. We'll discuss antibiotics and their use and misuse in greater detail in Chapter 3 along with probiotic options to reduce the harmful side effects of antibiotic drugs.

Chapter 2

The Surprising Worlds Within Your Body

"Life on earth is such a good story you cannot afford to miss the beginning . . . beneath our superficial differences we are all of us walking communities of bacteria. The world shimmers, a pointillist landscape made up of tiny living beings."

—Lynn Margulis, American biologist and professor,
University of Massachusetts, Amherst

Wes Battles Cancer Naturally

Wes, a sixty-two-year-old farmer, drove four hours each way to see me, explaining he wanted a natural approach for the stomach cancer he had recently been diagnosed with. As a soft-spoken gentleman, Wes quickly became one of my favorite clients, although his challenging health circumstances meant we had to use a heavy-handed approach. Stomach cancer is frequently terminal, so I knew we had to use the best tools in the natural medicine arsenal.

Wes Battles Cancer Naturally (continued)

He told me that the doctors gave him less than a year to live, something that always bothers me considering I've seen many people live much longer than doctors predict. I too am one of these people, considering I wasn't "supposed" to live beyond twenty-one. So I felt a kinship with Wes and wanted to do everything I could to help him fight cancer.

I put Wes on a diet rich in anticancer foods like garlic, onions, hempseeds, fish oils, leafy greens, legumes, beets, blackberries, broccoli, cabbage, tomatoes, and turmeric along with fermented foods like sauerkraut, kimchi, vegan yogurt, and others. I knew from experience with a wide range of clients that these foods support the body in restoring health, and I believed they could strengthen Wes so his body was as strong as possible to fight cancer. I also asked him to avoid sugar and alcohol, as many cancers feed on sugar.

I asked him to take a high-dose probiotic that included *Bifidobacterium lactis*, or what I call the "antitumor superhero"; *Streptococcus thermophilus*, the gene genie; and *Lactobacillus brevis*, "the booster of anticancer compounds," as the latter had been shown to boost the body's production of anticancer compounds, known as interferon, in research. I was aware that these probiotics had been effective against cancer in research and hoped they would have the same outcome with Wes. Additionally, the formula I selected also contained *B. longum*, *L. salivarius*, *L. rhamnosus*, and *L. plantarum*, as these probiotics have a history of aiding nausea and inflammation and help restore beneficial bacterial imbalances in the body.

Because Wes needed a full program to support his fight against cancer, I asked him to take an herbal formula known as Essiac, which was originally used by the First Nations people of Canada as a natural anticancer remedy and later passed down to a nurse who commercialized the product. I added an enzyme that destroys many free radicals, compounds that damage cells and can lead to cancer, and superoxide dismutase along with curcumin, which is an extract of the spice turmeric and has demonstrated anticancer properties in research. To help keep his energy strong so he could battle the cancer, I recommended ginseng.

He came back to see me every month and made biweekly calls to report on his progress, which for the first several months seemed nonexistent. Then he came to see me, grinning from ear to ear. His latest scan had shown a significantly smaller tumor. It wasn't gone, but we were both thrilled to see improvement of any kind, considering his prognosis. Wes continued to battle the cancer with all the natural medicines I recommended along with the chemotherapy and radiation treatments his medical doctor prescribed. He fought long and hard, and finally, after about thirteen months, he came to see me and shared that his MD didn't know how it was possible, but there was no sign of the tumor. I couldn't have been happier. Although I wish this was the case for every person with terminal cancer, unfortunately it isn't. But I rejoiced that Wes was alive and well. He was worn out from the battle, but he won his war on cancer.

The Landscape of Tiny Living Beings

You may believe that you are a collection of organs, bones, and tissues and that you are the single unifying consciousness between all of these body parts. But you are so much more than that and perhaps more than you are even aware of. Your body is the landscape upon which approximately 100 trillion bacteria live. Your body actually contains more bacteria than human cells. The average person has 100 trillion bacteria and between 50 to 100 trillion human cells. That may sound scary but without bacteria you could not exist—you need them to live.

For your hospitality in sharing your life and body with these beneficial bacteria, they contribute to the many aspects of your health and your survival. They fight disease for you, ensure the digestion of your food, manufacture nutrients that you need to form healthy cells and tissues, and kill nasty intruders that intend you harm. They attempt to reduce or eliminate any pain you may experience and even regulate the production of compounds in your body that stabilize your mood so you feel as good as possible and be free of anxiety or depression.

Making friends with these microscopic inhabitants within and encouraging their survival is the key to your great health and resistance to disease. As we learn more and more about probiotics we discover that disease or ill health tends to strike when we, knowingly or unknowingly, do things that upset our body's natural balance of bacteria. And although eating some yogurt daily may be a single step in the right direction, it is only one step. What's more, depending on the yogurt you choose, it might actually do more harm than good, but I'm getting ahead of myself here. I'll explain more momentarily.

Once you understand some of the cast of bacteria upon which your health depends you will realize that one of the greatest ways to transform your health is to encourage certain microorganisms to thrive within your body. How can you do that? Keep reading and you'll soon learn the many ways to support the beneficial bacteria within your body so they will repay you with the great health you deserve. Later in this chapter and throughout the next few chapters of *The Probiotic Promise* I'll introduce the cast of bacteria in detail and explain their many functions in your body as well as the exciting research that is demonstrating their effectiveness against so many different health conditions.

The Good, the Bad, and the Undetermined

Perhaps you've heard that there are harmful bacteria in your intestines. If so, you've heard right. You may also have heard about good bacteria being at war with the harmful ones to keep them in check. Although this is somewhat true, it is not actually the whole story. Dr. Hiromi Shinya, MD, a gastroenterologist with over fifty years' experience studying intestinal bacteria, diet, and the link between them, found that the intestinal bacteria go beyond the concept of good vs. evil. He discovered that

> The proportion of bacteria in our intestines is approximately 20 percent beneficial bacteria, 30 percent harmful bacteria, with the remaining 50 percent being intermediate bacteria. The key bacteria that contribute to the control of the intestinal environment are the intermediate bacteria. This is so because, when the proportion of harmful bacteria increases as the result of irregular meals and other bad eating habits, intermediate bacteria are drawn into the domain of harmful bacteria and the majority of intestinal bacteria act as harmful bacteria, decomposing undigested foods and generating toxic gas.[1]

Essentially, it is like the intermediate bacteria in our intestines are subject to peer pressure from the beneficial or harmful bacteria, and our food choices affect them even further. Although this may sound scary, it is actually empowering. It means that we have a significant amount of control over our health. It means not only that our dietary and lifestyle choices can dramatically increase the 20 percent of beneficial bacteria we have in our intestines but also that these choices can help sway the intermediate bacteria to our side. Dr. Shinya describes these intermediate bacteria as the "swing voters," as they are undecided as to join the camp of good or evil.

When it comes to the intestines, what happens there plays a significant role in the health of your whole body. So getting the "swing voter" bacteria on the side of the good bacteria while at the same time increasing the numbers of the healthy bacteria can mean the difference between great health or poor health. Some health conditions caused by gluten intolerance, including celiac disease or gluten sensitivity, can actually give the harmful pathogens advantages and shift the intestines' conditions in their favor, which can lead to bloating or even serious intestinal conditions beyond the original one. Later I'll share more information on how your intestinal health plays a role in determining the health of your whole body. I recall one of my earliest nutrition textbooks, almost twenty-five years ago, which was written by a wise man and health pioneer, Dr. Bernard Jensen, who wrote about the importance of the intestines to overall health. He was obviously ahead of his time, and science is now discovering that what he said was true. In my two and a half decades of experience working with thousands of clients I can say with confidence that intestinal health *is* the secret to overall health and wellness.

Your intestines are not the only place in the body where probiotics reside. Let's explore the bacterial landscape further.

Our Internal Ecosystems

You may think that you are only you. After all, what else could you be? But in the same way that scientists have been busy cataloging DNA in the Human Genome Project, other scientists are busy cataloging the many bacteria that live on or within the human body in the Human Microbiome Project (HMP). They found that each human being has a collection of ecosystems in various parts of his or her body. We have ecosystems in our intestines, in our mouth, on our tongue, on our teeth, on the front of our knees, on the back of our knees, on our nose, on our wrists, on our left hand, on our right hand, and on and on. You get the picture.

Scientists refer to the *microbiome* as the communities of microorganisms that inhabit your skin, mouth, gut, and other parts of your body.[2] Although the research to catalog the microorganisms on humans is ongoing, so far scientists have discovered that a person's left hand varies significantly from her right hand; only 17 percent of the bacteria on a person's left and right hands will be similar.[3] And your right hand likely differs significantly from mine. We know from experience that our fingerprints differ from every other human on the planet; we are also learning that no two microbiomes are the same. The collection of bacteria inhabiting our body is a product of our life experience and unique to us.

Scientists working on the HMP are exploring the ecosystems within our bodies in five sites on the human body, including nasal passages, oral cavities, skin, gastrointestinal tract, and urogenital tract.[4] Although many other ecosystems exist, they are currently focusing their efforts to catalog the microbes in these areas. With trillions of bacteria residing in our bodies, the magnitude of their project is vast. Only a matter of years ago we considered the Human Genome Project to catalog human DNA to be one of the greatest scientific achievements of our time. From the sheer amount of cataloging necessary to complete the Human Microbiome Project, it will surpass the magnitude of the Human Genome Project. At this point bacteria isolated in the HMP are not being studied for their health-promoting or health-destroying characteristics, just for whether they appear to be "normal" between different people. Over time their focus may shift, but for now developing a catalog of the many different types of microbes that

The *New York Times* recently reported on the microbiome from different journalists' perspectives. My favorite piece was "Some of My Best Friends Are Germs," in which Michael Pollan, best-selling author of *The Omnivore's Dilemma*, described his life: "I can tell you the exact date that I began to think of myself in the first-person plural—as a superorganism, that is, rather than a plain old individual human being." He proceeded to share his experience of getting his microbiome sequenced by the BioFrontiers Institute at the University of Colorado, Boulder. It wasn't the part about the microbiome sequencing that fascinated me, although it was fascinating in its own right; it was his recognition that the new science that our bodies contain countless bacteria was not something to be feared as disgusting but rather to be exalted because we are so much more miraculous than we ever dreamed possible, that we are not simply individuals but rather whole ecosystems and that countless other living beings rely on us and depend on us for their very existence—and that we depend and rely on them as well for ours. This realization is exciting and enormous.

inhabit our bodies offers insight to our bodies we have not yet explored. This will lead to a greater understanding of our bodies and how they interact with the larger world as well as insights into how to restore balance and overcome illness. I can't wait to see what these scientists continue to discover, as I'm sure it holds huge promise for the future of healing.

What's All the Fuss About Gut Health Anyway?

What happens in your gut plays a significant role in determining the health of your whole body. Your gut plays a critical role in the health of your brain, joints, respiratory system, and much more. It is a factor in whether you'll experience allergies or have a healthy immune system. Although more and more people are talking about gut health, it's usually not in the context of our health beyond the gut. But there is good reason to start considering gut health as a key factor in maintaining or restoring great health throughout your body.

Your body contains trillions of microorganisms. Although microorganisms exist throughout the body, they are primarily stationed in the intestines. Over 1 trillion bacteria made up of an estimated one thousand different species reside in your intestines.[5] The microbes in your body weigh an estimated two pounds.

The presence of beneficial bacteria in the gut are integral to the health of your GI tract, which in turn plays a significant role in determining the health of your whole body, from the brain in our head down to the smallest joints in our toes. As you learned in the last chapter, it is essential to have sufficient probiotic bacteria in the intestines not only to perform their many functions but also to sway the intermediate bacteria to act as beneficial bacteria. Probiotics aid digestion, ensure the proper absorption of essential nutrients, eliminate waste products from the intestines, aid the manufacture of critical vitamins, control harmful bacteria and other microbe populations in the body, quell inflammation, regulate the immune system, metabolize excess cholesterol, and perform other necessary functions.

When it comes to quelling inflammation in the body and regulating the immune system, probiotics truly are superstars. Conversely, insufficient probiotics or excessive harmful microbes in the intestines can create inflammation and result in an unbalanced immune system, as is especially the case with autoimmune diseases. Research shows that probiotic bacteria are far more intelligent than we may have realized. They can recognize the disease-causing molecular patterns of harmful microbes and respond by secreting proteins that destroy the harmful microbes.[6] The beneficial probiotics also secrete anti-inflammatory compounds that affect the walls of the intestines, which helps to regulate the immune system and prevent overactive responses to the environment, as in the case of allergies, or to the body's own tissues, as in the case of autoimmune disorders.

So how do you know that your bowel flora are out of balance? Stool samples taken by doctors or laboratories don't measure probiotics, but they can measure specific harmful infectious bacteria and yeasts that may be present in your intestines. Typically, however, a doctor may suspect a specific infection, perhaps *E. coli*, and he or she will order a lab test to determine whether you have that infection. The lab doesn't screen for all possible harmful microbes in a single stool sample—that's just not possible. So although these types of tests are definitely helpful in determining certain types of infections, keep in mind that they present limited information. Of course, if you suspect an intestinal infection, I highly recommend working with a physician to obtain relevant laboratory tests to help you assess what's happening. The Resources section on page 241 of this book identifies some diagnostic tests that may help your physician determine underlying factors that may be affecting your health.

An imbalance of harmful bacteria to beneficial probiotics in the intestines tends to cause uncomfortable symptoms, so assessing these symptoms can be helpful in determining whether you have an underlying imbalance. Of course, it's not fool-proof, so it should only be considered a general guide.

Some of the signs of an intestinal overgrowth of harmful bacteria or yeasts include:[7]

abdominal pain or cramping

acid reflux and heartburn

acne

allergies and food sensitivities

anxiety

any disorder of the digestive tract

autoimmune disorders (rheumatoid arthritis, lupus,
    Hashimoto's thyroiditis, fibromyalgia, etc.)

back pain

bad breath, gum disease, and dental problems

belching

bloating

chronic fatigue

constipation

diarrhea

difficulty losing weight

diverticulitis/diverticulosis

eczema or psoriasis

fibromyalgia

flatulence

high cholesterol

indigestion

irritable bowel syndrome

joint inflammation and stiffness

nausea

poor digestion

poor sleep

sinus infections

sugar cravings

yeast infections or vaginitis

This list is by no means exhaustive. Many different seemingly unrelated health conditions can be linked to poor bowel health. Constipation or fewer than one bowel movement daily is linked to disease. The medical journal *Lancet* published a study in which scientists found a link between poor intestinal health and breast disease.[8] Women who had daily bowel movements had fewer incidences of breast disease than those who didn't, and women who had two or fewer bowel movements weekly had four times the likelihood of breast disease. Additional research in the *American Journal of Public Health* found an increased incidence of breast cancer among women who had infrequent bowel movements, hard stools, or constipation.[9] In the next two chapters you'll discover many other health problems linked to poor intestinal health or overgrowth of harmful intestinal microbes and/or a deficiency in probiotic bacteria and, more importantly, how probiotics are showing great promise as a preventative measure and therapeutic aid.

Candida—The Silent Epidemic

There are many kinds of opportunistic infections that can inhabit our intestines. One of the most common is known as *Candida albicans*, which is a type of fungus but is commonly referred to as a yeast infection. Jacob Teitelbaum, MD, author of *From Fatigued to Fantastic*, found that yeast overgrowth is linked to an average weight gain of 32.5 pounds per person.[10] And, according to some estimates, at least 15 million women suffer from candidiasis, the condition caused by an overgrowth of the fungus Candida. But Candida really doesn't discriminate based on gender; men are vulnerable to its effects as well. The following list notes some of the most common symptoms of candidiasis.

Common Symptoms of Candida[11]

General—chronic fatigue, sweet cravings, weight gain, skin conditions (acne, eczema, psoriasis)

Gastrointestinal system—thrush, bloating, gas, intestinal cramps, rectal itching, alternating diarrhea and constipation

Genitourinary system—vaginal yeast infections, frequent bladder infections

Hormonal system—menstrual irregularities, PMS, menopausal symptoms, fibroids, endometriosis

Nervous system—depression, irritability, trouble concentrating, brain fog

Immune system—allergies, chemical sensitivities, lowered resistance to infections, arthritis

There are at least 150 species of fungi that are collectively known as Candida, but *Candida albicans* is one of the most frequently overgrown. It releases over eighty known toxins that weaken the body's defenses and cause the gut's membranes to become increasingly permeable, which allows undigested protein molecules to pass across intestinal walls and absorb into the bloodstream. A host of different health conditions, including allergies, food and chemical sensitivities, fibromyalgia, rheumatoid arthritis, and many other diseases, can result. I'll further discuss this condition, known as leaky gut syndrome, momentarily.

What causes the overgrowth of Candida or other microbes in the intestines? There are many factors, including:

• Alcohol intake (wine, beer, liquor): Many harmful microbes feed on the alcohol and sugars found in these beverages, which can lead to an overgrowth of harmful microbes. Beer is especially an issue because of its maltose content. Maltose is a sugar that feeds yeasts and some bacteria.

- Antacid use: Using commercial antacids can actually deplete your body's hydrochloric acid production (more on this below), which works as the body's first line of defense against many harmful microbes, giving them an opportunity to take hold in the body.
- Antibiotic use: Antibiotics destroy many harmful bacteria and beneficial ones alike, giving the harmful ones, especially those that have developed antibiotic resistance, an opportunity to overgrow.
- Birth control pills: Birth control pills are comprised of the hormone estrogen. This synthetic form of estrogen has been shown to promote the growth of fungi and affect intestinal bacteria.[12]
- Blood sugar imbalances: When blood sugar rises, it feeds harmful microbes. When blood sugar falls, we tend to crave sweets and refined carbohydrates that also feed harmful microbes, thereby causing beneficial bacteria in the gut to decline and the harmful ones to take hold.
- Chlorinated water consumption: Chlorine kills bacteria in our municipal water systems, but it also kills beneficial gut flora. Most tap water contains chlorine.
- Consumption of foods that contain antibiotics and synthetic hormones (nonorganic chicken, dairy products, and meat).
- Diabetes: Diabetes is linked to high blood sugar levels, which can allow pathogenic organisms to grow unchecked and make it more difficult to contain infections.
- Excessive sugar intake: Harmful, infectious microbes feed on sugar, giving them an opportunity to propagate at the expense of your health.
- Hypothyroid function: A low thyroid function can be a factor in compromising digestion and the immune system, and this can cause a reduction in probiotics and an increase in harmful bacteria and fungi.
- Immunosuppressive drugs (steroids, cortisone, etc.): These drugs not only interfere with your body's immune system that would

normally fight off pathogenic microbes but also cause imbalanced blood sugar levels that give these harmful microbes an opportunity to proliferate.

- Insufficient hydrochloric acid production: Hydrochloric acid is naturally produced by the stomach and acts as one of the first lines of defense against harmful microbes like those that cause food poisoning. Insufficient hydrochloric acid also causes incomplete digestion, which can result in the fermentation of carbs, and this feeds many pathogenic bacteria and fungi. Medications that lower stomach acid can also contribute to the problem.
- Mercury amalgam dental fillings: The silver fillings in your mouth are made up of at least 50 percent mercury, which is largely released as vapors into your body. Mercury kills beneficial bacteria, thereby allowing harmful microbes to take hold.
- Multiple sexual partners or sex with an infected person: Some infectious diseases, including yeast infections, can be spread through sexual contact.
- Nutritional deficiencies: Dietary deficiencies of vitamins, minerals, amino acids, and essential fatty acids aid harmful microbial overgrowth. Without these nutrients, the body's immunity may be compromised.
- Poor diet: A diet high in sugars and refined carbohydrates (think pastries, cookies, cakes, doughnuts, white bread, and pasta) feed harmful microbes, giving them an opportunity to take hold.
- Recreational drug use: Many drugs damage the digestive tract and kill beneficial probiotic bacteria.
- Stress, particularly ongoing, chronic stress: Stress causes the adrenal glands, two triangular-shaped glands that sit atop the kidneys, to release the hormone cortisol, which, over time, can depress the immune system and cause a rise in blood sugar, the latter of which feeds harmful microbes.

- Toxic exposures: In addition to mercury, other toxic metals can kill beneficial bacteria, allowing harmful microbes to take hold. Many toxins from plastics, known as xenoestrogens, also act like potent estrogens in the body and can promote the growth of harmful bacteria and fungi in the intestines.
- Weakened immunity: A compromised immune system can allow harmful microbes to grow in the body without the normal immune response. Conversely, an imbalanced ratio of harmful to beneficial bacteria in the intestines can also weaken immunity.[13]

Candida, and possibly other harmful microbes, also produces hormone-like substances that interfere with normal hormone production. These hormone-like substances can disrupt the body's normal hormone balance, especially in women. Additionally, studies suggest that Candida overgrowth is likely an underlying factor in some allergic reactions and for the increase in allergies over the past few decades.[14]

By now you may have realized that such a discussion in a book on probiotics and fermented foods must mean they can help—and you'd be right. Restoring healthy gut balance with probiotic-rich foods along with high-quality supplements can help destroy Candida and reduce any negative symptoms associated with it. Candida can really only take hold if we have an intestinal bacterial imbalance in the first place, so restoring the balance is the first (and best) step toward getting Candida under control.

Do You Have the Guts for Great Health?

Before we can experience great overall health we must restore GI health to reduce inflammation in the body, now linked to almost every chronic health condition ranging from arthritis to cancer, and to ensure healthy immunity to disease. To understand the gut link to inflammation throughout the body, it will be helpful to first take a brief tour of the gastrointestinal system.

Your Gastrointestinal System

The digestion process is actually transformative, yet most people never give it a second thought until some uncomfortable symptom occurs. The food you eat contains protein, carbs, and fats, all of which need to be broken down into amino acids, sugars, and fatty acids, respectively. These are some of the building blocks of every cell, tissue, and organ in your body. Ideally the food you eat also contains vitamins, minerals, and many other components such as enzymes, phytonutrients, and probiotics. I still regularly hear someone state that "vitamins aren't necessary," but actually they are. The Oxford Dictionary definition of *vitamin* is "any of a group of organic compounds which are *essential* for normal growth and nutrition and are required in small quantities in the diet because they cannot be synthesized by the body."[15] Minerals are the inorganic substances found in food that are essential to the functioning of the body, such as calcium, magnesium, iron, and others.

The GI system comprises many organs, including the mouth, salivary glands located in the mouth, stomach, small intestine, large intestine, liver, gall bladder, pancreas, and others, but these are the main ones we'll discuss. The average person's GI tract is about twenty feet long, processes approximately twenty-five tons of food over a person's lifetime, and serves many other functions in our body.

When you eat food, digestion immediately begins in your mouth through the act of chewing. While you are busy chewing to break down the food, your salivary glands begin to secrete digestive juices full of enzymes that further break down the food, particularly starches and sugars. If you are busy working, driving, or engaged in conversation during mealtimes and not adequately chewing your food, you're actually minimizing a critical step in digestion, both because food won't be broken down sufficiently and because it won't adequately mix with salivary enzymes.

Once you swallow the food it passes down through a tube known as the esophagus until it reaches the stomach. In the stomach the food sits for about twenty to thirty minutes, mixing with any enzymes within the food (uncooked foods only) and with the salivary enzymes, which further break down the food. At that point the food, particularly ones high in protein, sustain an *acid bath* as they mix with hydrochloric acid secreted by the stomach.

The food then passes into the small intestines, where nutrients are absorbed through villi in the intestinal wall and pass directly into the bloodstream. *Villi* are fingerlike protrusions that help absorb nutrients from food more efficiently. Water and essential nutrients are extracted, allowing these nutrients to absorb through the walls of the intestines directly into the bloodstream, where they will travel to the places they are most needed. For example, calcium frequently travels through the intestinal walls into the blood and then to the bones, muscles, nerves, or other parts of our body that need calcium to function properly.

Our bodies depend on many vitamins and minerals that are necessary as the building blocks of cells. A single nutrient deficiency can cause a host of problems in the body. That is one of the reasons why maintaining healthy small intestines is critical for good health. I'll explain other reasons momentarily.

The liver, which sits below your lower ribcage on the right side of your body, produces a greenish-colored substance called bile and sends it to the gallbladder for storage and secretion as needed to assist with breaking down fatty foods. The gallbladder secretes this bile, which starts the contractions of the intestines to push any waste matter left after the water and nutrients have been extracted from food out of your large intestines.

Now consider that the Standard American Diet, deservedly also called SAD, is deficient in vitamins, minerals, other plant nutrients, water, and fiber. It is also high in sugar, artificial chemicals and preservatives, and inflammation-causing fats as well as having a host of other nutrition issues. This diet wreaks havoc on the intestinal walls by the fingerlike villi protruding from the gut wall. Not only do the damaged villi become less capable of absorbing nutrients from our food and supplements; they can also become inflamed from the damage and can even change shape over time, which further affects their ability to perform their nutrient-extraction responsibilities.

Damaged and inflamed intestinal walls lead to an upset in the normal balance of beneficial to pathogenic microbes, which is called *dysbiosis*. This imbalance can further allow harmful bacteria and yeasts to multiply, causing a host of negative symptoms depending on the type of infections present. Dysbiosis can cause increased permeability of the intestinal walls, making it easier for harmful microbes to hijack the nutrient-absorption process and instead allow waste products and pathogenic microbes direct access to the bloodstream.

Although medical scientists continue to search for the cause or causes of autoimmune disorders—those in which the body attacks its own tissue—of which there are over eighty, including conditions such as rheumatoid arthritis, celiac disease, lupus, and multiple sclerosis, I believe dysbiosis is one of the primary causes of autoimmune diseases and a range of other illnesses.[16] I also believe that dysbiosis is an underlying factor for many other health conditions. Reinstating a healthy diet, healing the gut, and restoring a healthy balance of beneficial-to-pathogenic microbes is essential in addressing most illnesses. Restoring beneficial microbes helps to defend our bodies against harmful bacteria, viruses, yeasts, parasites, inflammatory disorders, and even the damaging effects of drugs like antibiotics.

The Gut-Inflammation Connection

More and more research shows that inflammation is a root cause of most diseases and is frequently the result of excessive numbers of harmful microbes and insufficient numbers of probiotic microbes in the intestines. When this happens you may be experiencing silent inflammation without even realizing it. Worse than that, it may be stealing your health without your awareness. An increasing amount of research links inflammation to fibromyalgia, chronic fatigue, arthritis, cancer, heart disease, diabetes, obesity, and many other health concerns.[17] Yet few people ever consider their gut health as a causal factor in these serious and debilitating health conditions. More often people assume that some of these illnesses are simply the signs of aging. But even some of the signs of aging that we consider inevitable may actually be the result of "wear and tear" from our poor eating habits and lifestyle patterns over a lifetime or from the changes in bacteria in our gut over time.

Research shows that aging is linked to marked reductions of several important probiotic species, especially the Bifidobacteria and Bacteroides.[18] A reduction in these beneficial bacteria can set the stage for improper immune sensing by the lymphoid tissue in the gut, also known as *gut-associated lymphoid tissue* (GALT), which leads to increased inflammation and intestinal permeability, frequently referred to as "leaky gut syndrome." When this happens the body responds by increasing the production of many inflammatory proteins that keep not only the gut inflamed but can also cause inflammation that can spread anywhere in the body.[19] So you could experience aches and pains in your fingers or perhaps your knees, and you may not realize it could stem from your intestines.

Your body may be able to deal with the inflammation in the short term, but when the inflammation reaches a sufficient level many disease conditions may result, including heart disease, liver or kidney dysfunction, autoimmune conditions, neurological diseases, obesity, insulin resistance, type 2 diabetes, and many infectious diseases. Well-known vascular and cancer surgeon Dr. Leonard Smith adds that "it is interesting to note that HIV and aging share cellular immunologic similarities."[20] And, according to new research that I'll share in the next chapter, the body's microbial imbalance sets the stage for the symptoms of aging and vulnerability to diseases like HIV.

Sufferers of serious illnesses are not the only ones who may be experiencing low-grade inflammation and imbalanced intestinal flora thanks to our modern lifestyles, with little fresh food and an abundance of sugar-loaded, additive-filled, and overprocessed foods. Additionally, our high animal-protein diets, with few plant-based foods, can further imbalance our gut flora and lead to subclinical inflammation devoid of symptoms. Then add a course or two of antibiotics, birth control pills, over-the-counter pain medications, or other drugs that further damage the microbiome, and you are left vulnerable to infections and other health concerns.

If you suspect that your intestinal flora are unbalanced, you may be wondering what you can do to kill harmful pathogenic microbes in the intestines, replenish the probiotics, heal damage to the intestinal walls, and quell inflammation that starts in the intestines. Many of the conditions linked to gut bacterial imbalances and excessive intestinal permeability can be corrected with

The Leaky Gut Link

Some members of the medical community are reluctant to recognize that an increased number of pathogenic bacteria and insufficient beneficial microbes can lead to increased permeability of the intestines, also known as *leaky gut syndrome*. Leaky gut is a condition in which the intestinal walls become increasingly permeable, allowing intestinal contents such as bacteria, viruses, toxins, food particles, or intestinal waste to travel across the wall to the bloodstream and making us vulnerable to inflammation, immune conditions, and many other health problems. But the evidence that leaky gut syndrome is a factor in many illnesses, particularly in immune conditions, is mounting.[21] Some of the symptoms of a leaky gut include bloating, cramps, fatigue, food sensitivities, flushing, achy joints, headache, and rashes. It can result in celiac disease, Crohn's disease, allergies, inflammatory bowel disease, ulcerative colitis, irritable bowel syndrome, arthritis, psoriasis, eczema, and asthma. Because it can give viruses access to the blood, it may set the stage for viral conditions like viral hepatitis and even HIV. It has also been linked to Alzheimer's disease.[22] Recent research in the *Journal of Alzheimer's Disease* and *PLoS One* found that the amyloid plaque formation in the brains of Alzheimer's victims is actually an antimicrobial compound made by the brain to fight viruses like the herpes simplex 1 and others.[23]

some dietary improvements, the regular addition of fermented foods, probiotic supplementation, and some other tweaks that restore our gut to a healthier state.

Eating more fermented foods and taking quality probiotic supplements are excellent ways to help restore the probiotic balance in our intestines. But as you'll learn in Chapter 6, not all fermented foods are created equally. Actually, our "go to" probiotic-rich food, yogurt, is surprisingly one of the lesser probiotic-rich foods. It's still a good choice when the cultures are alive, but you may be surprised to learn that there are many other fermented foods that are superior to yogurt at restoring gut health. Let's look a bit closer at how your diet plays a critical role in determining your overall health.

You Are What You Eat

The adage "you are what you eat" might never have been truer. According to new research your health may be determined by what you eat and what microorganisms come along for the ride. Although it may seem fairly obvious that a high-sugar diet would feed harmful disease-causing microbes that may reside in your intestines, it may surprise you to learn that other aspects of your regular diet may affect your gut health—like how much animal protein you eat. A new Harvard University study published in the journal *Nature* found that diet rapidly alters the microorganisms residing in the gut.[24] And if you eat a diet rich in meat or dairy products, you might not be happy with their findings. It has long been known that diet influences the type and activity of the trillion microorganisms residing in the human gut, but Harvard scientists found that even what we eat in the short term can have drastic effects on the type and numbers of microbes in our gut and their capacity to increase inflammation in the gastrointestinal tract.

The scientists discovered that microbes found in the food itself, including bacteria, fungi, and viruses, quickly colonized the gut. And, perhaps most notably, they discovered that an animal-based diet caused the growth of microorganisms that are capable of triggering inflammatory bowel disease within only two days of eating these foods. Still further research has linked inflammation-causing microbes to serious chronic diseases, meaning that the Harvard study has potentially far-reaching implications for disease prevention and treatment.

The scientists put volunteers on a meat-and-cheese diet, then switched them to a fiber-rich, plant-based diet to track the effect on intestinal microbes. They ate a breakfast of eggs and bacon, a lunch of ribs and briskets, and salami, prosciutto, and assorted cheeses for dinner, along with pork rind snacks. After a break from eating this diet, the volunteers ate a plant-based diet of granola for breakfast; jasmine rice, cooked onions, tomatoes, squash, garlic, peas, and lentils for lunch; and a similar dinner, with bananas and mangoes for snacks.

The scientists analyzed the volunteers' microbes before, during, and after each meal. The effects of the meat and cheese were immediate. The abundance of bacteria shifted about a day after the food hit the gut. After three days on either diet the bacteria in the gut also changed their behavior.

Lead scientist Lawrence David, PhD, admits that the meat-and-cheese diet used in his experiments was extreme; however, such an extreme diet helps to paint a clear picture of the outcome of a diet heavy in meat and cheese—and frankly, this is a typical diet for many people who use high-protein diets to lose weight or those eating the SAD. This high animal-protein diet clearly demonstrates the microbial impact of animal protein–rich diets. Dr. David said in an interview with *NPR*, an online journal, "I love meat . . . but I will say that I definitely feel a lot more guilty ordering a hamburger . . . since doing this work."[25] He also indicates that the study unlocks a potentially new avenue for treating intestinal disease. I would add that it likely unlocks ways to treat other inflammatory diseases in the body because heart disease, diabetes, arthritis, and even cancer have been linked to inflammation in the body.

What does this mean to you? Well, if you want to restore your gut and overall health, you may want to reconsider reaching for that bacon-wrapped sausage, cheese platter, or prime rib. Does that mean you have to become a vegan? Of course not—unless you want to. It means that heavy meat eaters would likely fare much better if they reduced their animal protein intake in favor of more plant-based options.

Few people even realize that there are many excellent plant-based sources of protein, so I shared my list here to help you make the switch.

Top Meat-Free Sources of Protein

High-protein diets like Atkins and South Beach have left many people thinking that animal products are the only options from which to get sufficient protein. That is simply not true. Most people eat excessive amounts of protein from these sources that, in addition to throwing off the delicate microbial balance in your gut, create high levels of acidity for their kidneys to address. Consider that our much thinner and healthier ancestors ate only about 5 percent of their caloric intake as animal protein, whereas we eat 40 percent of our calories as animal protein—that's a whopping 248 pounds of meat per person every year in the United States.

If you're looking to cut back on your meat, here are some vegan sources of protein you can include in your meals:

avocado

coconut

legumes, such as kidney beans, black beans, navy beans,
   pinto beans, Romano beans, chickpeas, soybeans,
   edamame (green soybeans)

nuts (preferably raw, unsalted), including almonds, Brazil nuts,
cashews, macadamia nuts, pecans, pistachios, and walnuts
(for my delicious probiotic-rich Savory Dairy-Free Greek-Style
Yogurt, see page 188)

quinoa

seeds, such as chia seeds, flaxseeds, hemp seeds, pumpkin seeds,
sunflower seeds, and sesame seeds

soy products (organic only, as soy is heavily genetically modified),
such as tofu, miso, and tempeh (for more on fermented soy
foods, see Chapter 5)

dairy alternatives, including almond milk, coconut milk, hemp seed
milk, and soy milk

You may notice that protein powders are not on the list. Although there are many excellent protein powders, there are also a significant number that are heavily processed, sugar-laden, or contain neurotoxic monosodium glutamate in one of its many guises, particularly as protein "isolates." If you are using protein powder, I recommend a high-quality hemp seed or pumpkin seed protein powder devoid of sweeteners and additives. Alternatively, add ground pumpkin, chia, flax, sunflower, or other types of seed to your smoothie as a great way to add protein, essential fats, and fiber to your diet. It's also a great way to feed beneficial microbes so they'll help strengthen your health against disease.

Meat is not the only food that causes a rapid change in the intestinal microbial environment. Research presented in the journal *Anaerobe* found that healthy adults who ate two apples daily for two weeks had significant changes in their number of probiotics in the stool, an indicator of the number of probiotics in the gut. The researchers found that after seven days of apple consumption the number of Bifidobacteria increased, and the number remained increased when the researchers reassessed the stool samples on day fourteen. They also found that the numbers of other probiotics like Lactobacillus and Enterococcus tended to increase. Keep in mind that no probiotics were actually administered in this study, so the increase in probiotics was based on existing probiotics in the gut proliferating. The scientists attribute the increase in microbes to the unique type of fiber found in apples, called pectin, as well as other apple components that still require research. Additionally, they found that the numbers of harmful pathogenic bacteria, such as *E. coli* and *Clostridium perfringens*, did not increase. In fact, the latter actually decreased, without any administration of anti-bacterial drugs or remedies. Simply adding apples to participants' diet was sufficient to reduce the harmful bacterial colonies.[26]

Build a Better Biome

B uilding a better microbiome in your body is not only one of the best ways to prevent health problems; it's also an excellent way to restore optimal health. The first step in building a healthier microbial balance is to improve your digestion. Here are some natural ways to improve your digestion, address harmful microbial infections, and swing the balance in favor of beneficial microbes.

Staying Regular for Great Health

Bowel health is not exactly what you would call a water cooler topic of conversation. Waste elimination is a private matter and often a private struggle for many people. Professional opinions vary on how many bowel movements an adult should have, ranging from three a day to three a week. I believe if you are not having

Strategies for Better Digestion

Here are some simple strategies to improve your digestion—and remember that great health starts with great digestion.

Avoid drinking much with meals. The liquid dilutes your body's natural digestive enzymes that are needed in full force to cope with all the heavy food most of us ingest. Limit your liquid intake with meals to less than a cup. If you're drinking with meals, choose fermented beverages like kefir or yogurt-based drinks.

Snack more and eat smaller meals throughout the day rather than eating huge meals. Your body is better able to digest food in smaller amounts.

Take your time. Chew your food well and really savor the taste by slowing down. Chewing mixes food with digestive enzymes that get started immediately to improve digestion. Remember our discussion about digestion: the stomach and intestines cannot do the job of the teeth, so make sure you chew well.

Eat earlier in the day and not too much just before bed. Your body needs adequate time for digestion. Lying down too soon afterward is a recipe for heartburn, indigestion, and poor nutrient absorption.

Try not to eat when you're feeling stressed out. If you're frequently stressed, try to create a more relaxing time to eat. Stress hormones send energy needed for digestion to other parts of your body and can result in indigestion.

Eat more fermented foods. Unpasteurized sauerkraut, yogurt, kefir, kimchi, or kombucha (a fermented tea beverage) are just a few examples of these delicious, health-promoting foods. The naturally present bacteria aid digestion and replenish the body's natural bacteria in the gut. You'll learn more about your many fermented food options in Chapter 6.

Supplement with a probiotic supplement on an empty stomach

upon rising in the morning. Choose a formula that contains a range of proven intestinal flora such as *Lactobacillus acidophilus* and *Bifidobacterium bifidus*. By regulating intestinal flora, you will also regulate bowel movements and improve digestion. (For more on how to sort through all the supplements out there, see Chapter 5.)

Supplement with a full-spectrum digestive enzyme product. It should contain a wide range of enzymes, as each one serves a unique purpose. Lipase aids fat digestion, protease aids protein digestion, amylase assists with carbohydrate digestion, lactase assists with digestion of dairy sugars, cellulase and hemicellulase assist with breaking down plant fiber.

Take apple cider vinegar for better digestion. If you struggle with digestion, start with a tablespoon of unfiltered, organic apple cider vinegar diluted in a half cup of water about ten minutes prior to eating your meals. The naturally fermented apple cider vinegar stimulates the body's natural production of hydrochloric acid to aid protein digestion. Avoid apple cider vinegar if you have been diagnosed with a stomach ulcer. However, many people who suffer from heartburn actually have insufficient hydrochloric acid.

Enjoy a peppermint or ginger herbal tea. Both have been shown in studies to improve digestion. Have them a few times during the day, though they are best drunk between meals rather than with meals, so wait at least an hour after eating to enjoy these delicious beverages. Instead of sugar, choose stevia, a sweetener that is naturally three hundred to one thousand times sweeter than sugar without having any impact on blood sugar or insulin levels.

Eat a largely plant-based diet and reduce your meat consumption. Meat and dairy products negatively affect the gut microbes within twenty-four hours of eating these foods. Eat more plant-based foods and protein sources (see page 39 for a list of these foods).

at least one or two healthy bowel movements a day, you may be suffering from constipation. If this becomes the norm, you may be suffering from chronic constipation, or your lack of regular elimination may be the symptom of another condition.

And if you recall our discussion about how nutrients and water are extracted from the food you eat, then you'll probably realize the importance of eliminating any fecal matter that may be backed up in your intestines before harmful toxins are absorbed into the bloodstream via this method. Additionally, being backed up can damage the delicate villi that line the gut wall, leaving you more susceptible to disease. When fecal matter gets backed up it can also contribute to an imbalance between the good and bad bacteria.

Backed-up bowels are common and can be caused by numerous factors. Insufficient insoluble fiber in the diet and not drinking enough water are the most common reasons people become constipated. The good news is that these issues are easy to fix by drinking more water and eating more high-fiber foods like vegetables, legumes, nuts, seeds, berries, and whole grains (unless your constipation is a symptom of Crohn's or colitis—additional fiber could make the condition worse). Irritable bowel syndrome (IBS) can also cause constipation, as can lack of exercise and the use of medications like pain killers. Temporary health changes like pregnancy can also result in temporary constipation.

If you have ruled out any underlying medical condition or pregnancy and are still not regular, here are some simple remedies to help boost your bowel function.

Probiotics—The Beneficial Bacteria. Take a full-spectrum probiotic supplement twice a day and well spaced from meals (try when you first wake up and when you are about to go to bed). These good bacteria are needed to manufacture healthy nutrients in the intestines, increase the absorption of vitamins, and control the proliferation of harmful bacteria. Don't be fooled by the commercials on television pushing yogurt and other processed foods as probiotic-rich solutions to your health issues. Although some yogurt is beneficial, there are many varieties of these products that have insufficient quantities and varieties of living cultures to do much good. Eat a wide variety of other fermented and cultured foods like those discussed in greater detail in Chapter 6 for the best results.

Magnesium. This mineral is an effective and gentle laxative that increases the water content in stools to support elimination. Most people eat a magnesium-deficient diet, which is easily corrected by adding dark leafy greens like spinach and kale, pumpkin and sesame seeds, cashews and almonds, and legumes and replacing red meat with fatty fish like wild salmon. A high-quality calcium-magnesium supplement, with at least 400mg of each mineral, is a good addition to your diet as well.

Aloe Vera. You don't hear much about aloe today, but the juice of this plant has been used for millennia to not only treat ulcerations in the digestive tract but also stimulate the elimination of fecal matter from intestines. A quarter cup of sugar-free, preservative-free aloe vera juice twice daily will help keep you regular.

Licorice Root. This medicinal herb tastes like many of the candies that bear its name but don't possess its therapeutic properties. Licorice root reduces inflammation in the intestines and helps eliminate waste. As an added bonus, a cup of licorice tea can help boost you when you are experiencing both emotional and physical stress. The herb is also available in tincture form. Individuals with high blood pressure or kidney failure as well as people taking heart medication should avoid licorice.

Yoga to Go. The yoga posture known as Apanasana is a simple and effective way to support intestinal cleansing and support the elimination of toxins. Throughout the day take a moment to stretch out on your back with your legs extended and arms down at your sides. Slowly lift your legs and bend your knees, drawing them toward your chest with your feet together and toes pointed away from you. Keeping your knees together over your chest, wrap your arms around your legs and hold for at least twenty seconds. Gently roll to your left and hold for twenty seconds, and then roll to your right and hold for the same amount of time. Repeat the entire process at least three times, and then relax on your back with your feet extended.

Colon Cleanse. If these other natural remedies and strategies are still not working, try a colon cleanse like the one I've outlined in detail in my book *Weekend Wonder Detox.*

The vast majority of people suffering from constipation can rid themselves of the problem—and the waste!—in a matter of days with a few simple lifestyle changes. If you don't see improvements after trying these tips and dietary changes, you may want to consult a qualified medical professional to determine whether the constipation is a symptom of an underlying health condition. However, most people will feel both regular and renewed with some simple lifestyle alterations.

Once you've set the stage for great health by improving your digestion and eliminating any constipation, you're ready to use probiotics for the many other health benefits they offer, from eliminating harmful disease-causing infections to boosting brain health and alleviating pain.

Chapter 3

From the Common Cold to Superbugs: Probiotics to the Rescue

"We mostly don't get sick. Most often bacteria are keeping us well."

—Bonnie L. Bassler, molecular biologist and professor, Princeton University

Angela Overcomes Chronic Fatigue

From the moment Angela awoke to the minute she climbed into bed, she was exhausted. She knew something was wrong, but the battery of medical tests hadn't found the source of her fatigue. When her medical doctor was quick to dismiss it, Angela knew she needed a different approach. That's when she came to see me.

Angela was only thirty-five when the fatigue set in after a series of stressful events in her life. When I asked her what was going on in her life just prior to the fatigue, she indicated that she had lost her job and took several months to find a new one, causing her to fall into a

Angela Overcomes Chronic Fatigue (continued)

pile of debt. Additionally, her best friend was diagnosed with cancer. Clearly Angela had been under a tremendous amount of stress that may have weakened her body. I ordered some tests, which showed she had a Candida infection along with weak adrenal gland function. The adrenals are two triangular-shaped glands that sit atop the kidneys and help the body cope with stresses of all kinds, including emotional stress, temperature fluctuations, altitude changes, excessive noise, physical traumas, and others.

We set straight to work on Angela's diet, which was heavy in hidden sugars and refined starches, not to mention the soda she drank on a regular basis. We eliminated all of these items at first to ensure that her diet was fairly sugar-free for at least a month. I recommended a probiotic supplement that contained strains with documented anti-inflammatory effects such as *L. bulgaricus*, *L. casei*, *L. plantarum*, *L. reuteri*, and *L. rhamnosus*. It also contained strains that had been shown to have antimicrobial effects, including *B. breve*, *S. thermophilus*, and especially *S. boulardii*, as the latter had demonstrated effectiveness against Candida infections in studies. Angela agreed to take two of the probiotic supplements three times daily.

I added some herbal antimicrobials like olive leaf and oregano oil, taken at least a few hours away from the probiotics to ensure they

We live in a germ-obsessed world and perceive bacteria as the enemy. Armed with antibacterial soaps, hand wipes, and cleaning products, we wage war against the perceived yet unseen enemy. Although it is true that some bacteria may be harmful or even deadly, there are countless bacteria that hitchhike their way through the world on our bodies and keep us healthy and alive in exchange for the ride.

didn't destroy the beneficial bacteria but instead went to work on the Candida infection. I included some ginseng, licorice root, and high doses of vitamin C to address the adrenal weakness.

Angela came back to see me in a month, reporting that her energy had definitely improved. She estimated that it was already 50 percent better than when I saw her a month earlier. I asked her to continue on the program I had created for her and to return in a month, which she did. At that time she reported feeling "back to herself" and felt she "could conquer the world." Although I was thrilled to hear it, I asked Angela to conserve a bit of that energy for her healing and to take time out for herself to prevent her adrenals from burning out. When I ran tests there was no sign of Angela's Candida infection and her adrenal function appeared normal. Angela is back on top of her life, feeling better than ever.

The Rise of Superbugs and the Fall of Antibiotics

For many years, beginning in the second half of the twentieth century, antibiotics became our primary weapon against bacteria-caused diseases and saved many peoples' lives in the process. Suddenly, we had incredibly effective medicines against bacterial illnesses, ranging from gonorrhea to pneumonia. And not only did antibiotics work; they worked quickly. With the help of antibiotics, we no longer had to worry that a cut or scrape was life threatening. After all, we had antibiotics. We no longer worried about most infectious diseases either because a quick trip to the doctor and a prescription for antibiotics could eliminate it in a matter of days.

But the overprescription of antibiotics, incorrect prescribing of antibiotics for viral illnesses, misuse of antibiotics, and overuse of antibacterial products has given harmful bacteria the opportunity to learn how to "outsmart" our best weapon against them—a whole class of drugs we call antibiotics.

Here's what happened: patients weren't happy leaving the doctors' offices without a prescription for a drug to alleviate their misery regardless whether they suffered from the common cold or a flu virus, so doctors handed them a seemingly harmless prescription for antibiotics. Remember: antibiotics only work on bacteria, not viruses!

At the same time and continuing through the present time, companies began manufacturing antibacterial soaps and cleaning products and air "fresheners" and disinfectants, scaring the public with images of creepy bacteria in commercials and advertisements so we would begin using these antibacterial products—and many people still do—with the hope that we'd avoid getting any of the colds and flu "going around." These products don't work on viruses either, and their effectiveness against other microbes is questionable as well, not to mention their toxic ingredients that are harmful to our health, but that's another story. (Check out my book *Weekend Wonder Detox* for more insight into the toxic story.) As a testament to our collective "germophobia," the Centers for Disease Control found that between 2003 and 2006 the toxic antibacterial substance found in many commercial soaps and sprays, triclosan, had increased in Americans' urine by 42 percent.[1] The increased amount of triclosan in our urine shows our increased exposure to this toxic antibacterial chemical.

Doctors also began overprescribing antibiotics for every bacterially linked condition, even for acne. I should know: by the time I was nine years old my doctor prescribed antibiotics that I was instructed to take for several *years*, just to treat adolescent acne. I'm not alone in this experience. Many other people received long-standing prescriptions for antibiotics to treat acne well before physicians' knowledge about the potential bodily damage outweighing any benefits of such a practice.

Veterinarians and factory farms also began overprescribing and misprescribing antibiotics for pets and farm animals as well. Some experts estimate that at least half of all antibiotics used in the United States go to huge factory farm operations.[2] Reporter Brandon Keim found that much of the antibiotic use "is used to treat diseases spread by industrial husbandry practices, or simply to accelerate growth. As a result, farms have become giant Petri dishes for superbugs, especially methicillin-resistant *Staphylococcus aureus* or MRSA, which kills twenty thousand Americans every year—more than AIDS."[3]

Those of us who took antibiotics for a bacterial illness often took them incorrectly too. We may have taken them for a few days, didn't notice any difference, so we stopped taking them altogether, even though the doctor advised taking the full prescription for a week or longer. Or we missed antibiotic doses thanks to our busy schedules, even though we should have followed the package.

Although we, our doctors, and antibacterial product manufacturers may have meant well, we collectively and inadvertently gave disease-causing bacteria the opportunity to become "educated" and learn how to outsmart antibiotic drugs. The idea of microscopic critters outsmarting some of our best medicines may seem outlandish, but it is exactly what has been happening since we first started using antibiotic drugs and antibacterial products. With the misuse, overuse, and abuse of our "miracle drugs," we created a monster and developed our current love-hate relationship with antibiotic drugs and the resulting fear of superbugs.

CBC News journalist Chris Wodskou describes the situation: "For the entire history of antibiotics, there's been an arms race of sorts between bacteria and medicine. Bacteria have developed resistance to one drug, and medicine has responded by producing new antibiotics. Bacteria develop resistance to the new ones, and medicine devises even newer antibiotics." But this is not a process that can continue indefinitely, as you'll soon discover, as the bacteria are discovering how to outsmart antibiotics they haven't even been exposed to yet. And the antibiotic approach is resulting in stronger and more virulent strains of bacteria. They're becoming like bacteria on steroids, in a way. He adds that "a lot of medical and public health experts now fear that we're on the cusp of an unsettling new age—the Post-Antibiotic Age."[4]

We have relied and continue to rely on antibiotics for so many things that most of us just take them for granted. Some of their uses include but are not limited to:

- addressing harmful bacterial infections;
- preventing wounds and injuries from becoming infected;
- helping organ transplant and chemotherapy patients whose immune systems have become vulnerable to infections; and
- using during or after surgery.

As if it weren't enough that bacteria are outsmarting our antibiotic drugs and antibacterial products, they are even sharing knowledge to help other bacteria outsmart them too. Stephen Harrod Buhner, author of *Herbal Antibiotics*, aptly described the situation: "Once a bacterium develops a method for countering an antibiotic, it systematically begins to pass the knowledge on to other bacteria at an extremely rapid rate. Under the pressure of antibiotics, bacteria are interacting with as many other forms and numbers of bacteria as they can. In fact, bacteria are communicating across bacterial species lines, something they were never known to do before the advent of commercial antibiotics. The first thing they share is resistance information and they do this in a number of different ways."[5]

Because we still use antibiotics heavily, many people who don't take the full prescription look for a way to get rid of any leftovers. That means people are flushing prescription leftovers down

How Bacteria Outsmart Antibiotics

Bacteria can share resistance information directly or by extruding it from their cells so that other bacteria can pick up the information at a later time. There are multiple ways bacteria share information on resistance, including:

- Encoding of plasmids, which are essentially DNA strands that are chromosome independent, to include resistance information, which they then pass on to other bacteria. These plasmids are highly mobile strands of genetic material that are widely exchanged among bacteria.
- Using transposons, parts of bacterial DNA that are sometimes called "jumping genes" because they allow a significant amount of resistance information to be released into the environment where other bacteria can later pick them up.
- Using viruses known as bacteriophages, or bacterial viruses, that make copies of the components of genes that contain resistance information and then spread to other bacteria.[6]

The commonly used antibiotic known as tetracycline has been shown to stimulate the transfer, mobilization, and movement of transposons and plasmids, by one hundred to one thousand times that of bacteria without exposure to tetracycline. This transfer of genetic material and information happens even with low doses of this antibiotic drug, which is a commonplace use of tetracycline.[7] This is just one example of how antibiotic drugs educate bacteria to become stronger and increasingly resistant to antibiotics. It's an excellent illustration of how bacteria don't just keep this newfound information to themselves; instead, they share it with other bacteria so they can collectively learn from the original bacteria's experience.

the toilet or are urinating them into the toilet—remember: if we take antibiotics, some of the drug will remain in our urine—all of which ends up in our water supply. Increasing numbers of reports are finding that the water supplies in most industrialized nations are contaminated with small amounts of antibiotics, meaning that water-borne bacteria are exposed to these antibiotics at low doses on an ongoing basis. Buhner says, "This exposure is exponentially driving resistance learning; the more antibiotics that go into the water, the faster the bacteria learn."[8]

Prior to the discovery and use of antibiotics we had no idea that bacteria, even different types, shared information to help them become stronger and multiply. Thanks to the advent of antibiotics we now know this to be true. Unfortunately, in the process we have encouraged the development of antibiotic-resistant bacteria. Few people would argue that antibiotics don't have merit; they have saved many lives and improved the quality of life for many people over the last century. But we are just beginning to understand the inherent problems of our misuse and overreliance on them: superbugs.

Creating Superbugs

As recently as 1970 people believed that scientists had outsmarted all infectious diseases. Surgeon General William Steward stated to Congress that "it was time to close the book on infectious diseases."[9] His statement represented what many people believed to be the situation. The discovery of antibiotics earlier that century had seemingly wiped out many infectious diseases of previous ages. But we are now discovering that many old diseases are coming back in a fiercer way.

According to the Centers for Disease Control and Prevention, "World health leaders have described antibiotic-resistant bacteria as 'nightmare bacteria' that 'pose a catastrophic threat' to people in every country in the world." In the United States alone every year at least 2 million people become infected with bacteria that are resistant to antibiotics. Sadly, an estimated twenty-three thousand of those people will die annually as a result of these infections.[10]

Consider MRSA as an example. The bacteria known as *Staphylococcus aureus* is now resistant to the antibiotic drug methicillin. That's how methicillin-resistant *Staphylococcus aureus* received its name, MRSA, for short. This disease once primarily infected immunocompromised individuals, or the very young and very old. Now healthy children and adults are also becoming infected with this bacterial infection. Although there are still antibiotics other than methicillin that can treat the disease that is linked to systemic infection of the blood, heart, spinal cord, or bones, some experts estimate that we are only a few years away from the disease having no antibiotic treatment at all.[11]

Experts also estimate that 30 percent of all *E. coli* urinary tract infections are resistant to treatment, whereas it was only 5 percent a decade earlier.[12] Possibly as a result of the growing concern about this bacterial infection, scientists have discovered that *E. coli* has developed a unique resistance method. Although *E. coli* and another bacteria known as Klebsiella were the first to use this form of resistance to antibiotics, many other disease-causing bacteria have since started using this particular mechanism to essentially disable our best antibiotic drugs. Essentially, *E. coli* and Klebsiella bacteria innovated new strategies to outsmart antibiotics.

This mechanism may have resulted in the infectious disease called carbapenem-resistant *Klebsiella pneumonia* (CRKP), which is an almost completely untreatable form of the bacterial infection Klebsiella that kills many of its victims. Another illness known as carbapenem-resistant *Enterobacteriaceae* (CRE) has also now emerged. The sexually transmitted disease gonorrhea is now seen

Extremely Scary Chicken Study

Every now and then I read a study that completely creeps me out. This is one of those studies. Once you read it I'm sure you'll understand why.

Studies like the one conducted by Stuart Levy, a professor who founded and runs the Levy Lab at the Center for Adaptation Genetics and Drug Resistance at Tufts University School of Medicine, may help us to further understand why antibiotic-resistant bacteria are on the rise. He conducted an experiment to follow the flow of resistant bacteria from farms. He took three hundred chickens and divided them into six groups of fifty per cage. Four cages were confined to a barn, while the remaining two were outside. Half of the chickens were given extremely low doses of the antibiotic oxytetracycline. Dr. Levy then assessed the feces of all the chickens and that of the families living nearby on a weekly basis.

Within twenty-four to thirty-six hours of eating the food containing the antibiotic drug the feces of all of the chickens that ate the food

as a serious threat, as the bacterial culprit has become resistant to antibiotic treatment. *Clostridium difficile* bacteria, which can cause symptoms ranging from diarrhea to life-threatening inflammation of the colon, have also become antibiotic resistant. The number of bacterial strains that are becoming resistant to what were once perceived as our best drugs is rapidly increasing.

Although most of us know that animals are given antibiotics, particularly on factory farms, we may be surprised to learn that they are sometimes used on produce as well. You read that correctly, I did state "antibiotics used on produce." In the United States, between forty and fifty thousand pounds of tetracycline and streptomycin are sprayed on fruit trees every year, primarily showed *E. coli*-resistant bacteria. Not long afterward, the chickens that never ate the antibiotic-containing food were also resistant to the drug. Shockingly, however, after three months the *E. coli* found in all of the chickens were resistant not only to the tetracycline but also to other antibiotics, including ampicillin, streptomycin, and sulfonamides, even though they never came in contact with these drugs. After six months their *E. coli* were resistant to an additional five antibiotics with which they never came into contact.

In a comparable German study researchers showed that in just over two years the people in the surrounding community also had antibiotic-resistant bacteria in their bodies.[13]

In an article published in the *New York Times*, "Gene Jumps to Spread a Toxin in Meat," infectious disease specialist Marguerite Neill stated, "In mankind's battle to conquer infectious diseases, the opposing army is being replenished with fresh replacements."[14]

on apple and pear trees to attack fire blight. Experts estimate that it is the equivalent of treating 18 million or more people with antibiotics.[15]

Farms are not the only places that may harbor antibiotic-resistant pathogens; hospitals have also become hot beds for antibiotic-resistant superbugs, such as MRSA, *C. diff*, and CRE.[16] Now patients are at risk of contracting these deadly diseases as a result of exposure to them while undergoing medical procedures in hospitals, many of which might have otherwise saved their lives.

It is imperative for our long-term health as individuals and especially collectively for future generations that we not only stop misusing antibiotics and antibacterial agents but also consider other options for keeping our immune systems strong and even for battling pathogenic bacteria. That's where probiotics come in.

Probiotics to the Rescue

Although fear may be the natural reaction to the situation we are now facing—and rightfully so—the story is not one of "doom and gloom"; it is actually one of hope and empowerment. Probiotics—the good bacteria—can help us in our battle against harmful bacteria and viruses, even antibiotic-resistant bacterial infections and superbugs. Exciting new research continues to stack up demonstrating the many ways probiotics are beneficial to our health and, more specifically, can help our bodies fight harmful infectious diseases. Although some of the research is preliminary, considering the safety and effectiveness that probiotics are demonstrating along with the seriousness of the situation we are facing, it is important to reveal our current and future ally in our effort to protect ourselves from harmful bacteria and improve our immunity against them.

Most people still view probiotic bacteria solely as beneficial for gut health, primarily to take alongside antibiotic drugs to prevent the side effects the drugs cause. Even regulatory agencies have restricted the claims that probiotic supplement manufacturers can make, only allowing digestion and immune health as claims even when the research demonstrating the therapeutic applications of probiotics goes well beyond the gut. And although probiotics are certainly beneficial for these purposes, they offer so much more than that in the possible treatment of other illnesses, even diseases that our best drugs can no longer stop.

Before we explore the mounting evidence that shows probiotics as a potential treatment for many serious or even deadly illnesses, let's first examine the way in which probiotics may work. New research suggests that probiotics may work in many different ways to help boost our immunity to disease and our overall health. Compare that with antibiotics, which work by indiscriminately killing all bacteria in their presence, good or bad—that

Some Probiotics Have Developed Resistance to Antibiotic Drugs

Because we discussed the antibiotic resistance of harmful pathogenic bacteria, you may be interested in knowing that some probiotics have also developed resistance to antibiotic drugs. Although the former situation can have deadly consequences for humans, the latter could actually be beneficial. Scientists at Guizhou University, the Chinese Academy of Sciences, Tsinghua University, and Renmin University of China collaborated on a study to assess one hundred strains of probiotic bacteria to determine whether they had also developed antibiotic resistance in their genes. They conducted tests on twenty-three substrains of *Lactobacillus delbrueckii bulgaricus*, twenty-six *Lactobacillus casei*, thirty *Streptococcus thermophilus*, five *Lactobacillus acidophilus*, six *Lactobacillus plantarum*, and ten *Lactobacillus paracasei*. The scientists found that all of the probiotics were resistant to the antibiotics gentamicin and streptomycin; forty-two were resistant to the drug vancomycin; and all were to some degree killed by the antibiotics cephalexin, erythromycin, tetracycline, and oxytetracline.[17] So what does this mean to you? It means that you'll want to replenish your supplies of probiotics when you're taking these specific antibiotics, as some still rampantly kill beneficial bacteria.

is, if the bacteria haven't developed a resistance to them. As we discussed earlier, an increasing number of bacterial strains are becoming resistant to antibiotics. But scientists know that probiotics are having many beneficial effects on our bodies. Here are nine ways they believe probiotics help boost our health:

1. They produce antimicrobial substances.
2. Probiotics improve the immune response to pathogens.
3. They decrease the inflammatory response in the body.

4. Probiotics assist in the early programming of the immune system to result in a better-balanced immune response and reducing the risk of the development of allergies.
5. They improve the mucosal barrier and its functions in the gut.
6. Probiotics enhance the stability and recovery of microbes in the body when they have been disrupted, through drugs like antibiotics, or poor food choices.
7. They regulate the gene expression for health conditions and diseases.
8. Probiotics create important proteins and enzymes the body needs.
9. They decrease the ability of pathogenic microbes from being able to adhere to locations in the body, such as the gut wall.[18]

Scientists propose these nine mechanisms as ways in which probiotics work even as they investigate these mechanisms in greater detail. While they continue to determine *how* they work, what they do know is *that* they work for many health concerns.

When the Medicine Is Worse Than the Illness

If you've ever taken a course of antibiotics, then you're probably familiar with some of the side effects of these drugs, including gastrointestinal distress, overgrowth of harmful bacteria in the intestines, and the resulting diarrhea. For many people the aftermath of taking antibiotics is as bad as the health problems that led them to take antibiotics in the first place. Fortunately, one of the areas in which probiotics truly shine is in dealing with harmful bacterial overgrowth and diarrhea that result from taking these drugs. Many doctors already advise patients to take probiotic supplements whenever they take antibiotic drugs. And that's for good reason. Research shows and many people have already experienced fewer drug side effects when they are taken in conjunction with probiotics. Scientists at DuPont Nutrition and Health, Kantvik Active Nutrition, in Finland, conducted a study to test the effectiveness of probiotic supplements to (1) prevent antibiotic-related diarrhea and (2) to assess the rate of C. *diff* infections and the resulting diarrhea from antibiotic use. They found that the higher the dose of probiotics, the lower the incidence and duration of diarrhea people experienced taking antibiotic drugs. They also found that participants taking probiotic supplements had fewer fevers, abdominal pain, and bloating.[19]

In another study of 255 adults, scientists gave some people two probiotic capsules containing *L. acidophilus* and *L. casei*, whereas others received one capsule of a placebo and one probiotic capsule, and still others received only placebo capsules. They found that the people receiving two capsules of probiotics daily had only half the incidence of antibiotic-associated diarrhea than those taking the one placebo and one probiotic and only one-third the incidence of the people taking only placebo pills. This study demonstrated not only that these two strains of probiotics worked to eliminate the side effects of antibiotic drugs but also that the higher the dose given, the better the results.[20] This study shows that when it comes to probiotics, size matters—dose size, that is. The scientists also concluded that timing plays an important role. When it comes to taking probiotics along with antibiotics, it is best to start taking probiotics right away and to continue taking them after completing the course of antibiotics.

Recently, researchers at the Beth Israel Deaconess Medical Center in Boston, Massachusetts, explored the large volume of studies linking probiotic use to the reduction in antibiotic-associated diarrhea. Their meta-analysis of thirty-four randomized, double-blind, placebo-controlled studies including 4,138 people found that probiotics taken with antibiotics prevent the antibiotic side effect of diarrhea.[21]

It's All in the Strains—Antibiotic-Associated Diarrhea

By now you may have also guessed that different strains of probiotics yield different results. You'll learn throughout this chapter and the next that although there is no single miracle strain that is effective against all illnesses, there are many strains that demonstrate tremendous effectiveness against specific conditions.

Lactobacillus plantarum is one strain of probiotic that works to cut the side effects of antibiotics.[22] Other research showed that *L. casei*, *L. bulgaricus*, and *S. thermophilus* also cut the incidence of antibiotic-associated diarrhea by almost two-thirds. This side effect may not seem like a big deal, but it is: diarrhea during or after antibiotic use demonstrates the rampant destruction of important intestinal bacteria, which can set the stage for other health conditions. Therefore, preventing it altogether is invaluable in the maintenance of good health and the prevention of disease. This kind of result is impressive by any standard, and when you consider that antibiotic-associated diarrhea can actually be quite serious and even life threatening, particularly among the elderly and immune-compromised individuals, this research demonstrates the potential for probiotics to improve health, reduce drug side effects, reduce health care costs, and even save lives.[23]

Some strains of probiotics have demonstrated effectiveness at reducing infections and diarrhea linked to antibiotics in infants and children, but not in adults. These strains include *Lactobacillus GG* and *Lactobacillus reuteri*.[24] That doesn't mean these strains are useless for adults, only that they were ineffective for adults with these symptoms

So we know that we have fewer side effects when taking probiotics alongside antibiotics, but what about probiotics' direct effects on harmful bacteria and infections resulting from them? This is an area where the research on probiotics is starting to shine.

in this study. In other studies *L. reuteri* has shown promise in treating side effects of chemotherapy in adult cancer patients, including diarrhea, as well as improving feeding tolerance in preterm infants. It also reduced the duration of hospitalization of preterm infants.[25] So don't make the mistake in thinking that *Lactobacillus reuteri*, or any other probiotic for that matter, is useless in all situations or even all cases of diarrhea. The message we can glean from this research is that we need to choose the best probiotic strains for our specific needs and circumstances, which we'll be discussing in great detail throughout the next couple of chapters.

Better Dental Health Through Probiotics

Periodontitis is a gum infection that damages the soft tissue in the mouth and can also destroy the bone that supports your teeth.[26] It can cause inflammation around the teeth and can result in pockets between the teeth and the gums. The disorder is, unfortunately, common and increases the risk of suffering a heart attack or stroke, so it is a good idea to address any possible infection as quickly as possible. Fortunately, some probiotics have also shown promise in treating dental disorders and can assist us with maintaining dental health.

A new study published in the *Journal of Clinical Periodontology* outlines findings on the effects of using lozenges containing the probiotic *Lactobacillus reuteri* over a twelve-week period on thirty otherwise healthy individuals who experienced periodontitis. The scientists ultimately found that subjects using the probiotic lozenges had a significantly greater reduction in the harmful bacteria linked to periodontitis as well as a significantly greater reduction in the depth of pockets around affected teeth. They also experienced a greater reduction in the bacteria known as a factor in the onset of chronic periodontitis.[27]

Healing Ulcers and Gastritis

Unfortunately, infection-related digestive system disorders are also common and becoming more worrisome, as the bacteria causing the infections are becoming increasingly resistant to the standard antibiotic treatment. Ulcers and gastritis are two common gastrointestinal conditions that are primarily linked with the overuse of nonsteroidal anti-inflammatory drugs (NSAIDs) or infection from the bacteria *Helicobacter pylori*.[28] Peptic ulcers are linked with painful sores or ulcerations in the stomach or upper intestines, whereas gastritis is an inflammation, irritation, or erosion of the stomach lining.[29]

Fortunately, as with many other bacterial infections, probiotics are showing promising results in treating *H. pylori* in both children and adults, reducing the side effects of drug treatment, as well as reducing the incidence of reinfection at a later date.

Several studies demonstrate that various strains of probiotic bacteria can inhibit the growth of *H. pylori*.

It's All in the Strains—H. Pylori Infections

In a Russian study researchers found that the probiotic *Bifidobacteria bifiform*, taken along with the standard drug treatment for *H. pylori*, improved the effectiveness of the drug treatment while also reducing the side effects of the drugs. The Russian scientists also found that the probiotics demonstrated antibacterial action and enhanced the body's own immune response against *H. pylori*.[30] Whereas the probiotics were used as an adjunct to drug treatment, the probiotics were effective against the condition as well.

If you're suffering from an *H. pylori* infection, which probiotic strains should you take? Some research shows *Bifidobacteria bifiform* is helpful.[31] In other studies that demonstrated the effectiveness of probiotics against *H. pylori* infections, scientists found that either Lactobacillus strains on their own or in combination with Bifidobacterium and Saccharomyces species effectively reduced the symptoms of *H. pylori* infection.[32]

How Probiotics Work

Because most of us don't give probiotics much thought, we may underestimate how powerful they are, especially against *H. pylori* bacteria. While scientists continue to study the role of probiotics in the treatment of ulcers, gastritis, and other gastrointestinal infections, they have found that probiotics appear to work against *H. pylori* bacteria and improve general gastrointestinal health in several ways. They believe that:

1. Bacteria in the Lactobacilli family help maintain bacterial balance.
2. Probiotic bacteria secrete various substances, known as bacteriocins, that may inhibit or destroy *H. pylori* bacteria. It may seem strange to think of probiotic bacteria as secreting antibacterial compounds, but when you consider that they are competing with other bacteria for food and space, it makes more sense.
3. Probiotic bacteria seem to prevent the ability of bacteria, including *H. pylori*, from adhering to the walls of the GI tract, thereby preventing the ability of *H. pylori* to survive.
4. Probiotics reduce inflammation by regulating the immune system's response to *H. pylori* bacteria (and others) and reducing inflammatory compounds.[33]

In several animal studies research shows that probiotic treatment effectively reduces the *H. pylori* infection and the gastrointestinal inflammation caused by the infection.[34] Although the studies haven't shown the ability of the probiotics used, in the dosages used in the studies, to completely eliminate the infection, neither have most of the drug studies either. Further research may help us determine whether a particular strain, combination of strains, in a certain dose, or in combination with another natural compound may be able to completely counter *H. pylori* infections. In fact, naturally occurring compounds found in cranberry juice have been shown in many studies to be effective against *H. pylori* infections; because of this, researchers conducted a study at the Laboratory of Microbiology and Probiotics, Institute of Nutrition and Food Technology, University of Chile, in Santiago, Chile, to assess the possible effects of combining cranberry juice with probiotics to treat *H. pylori* infections. The study shows the promise of treating *H. pylori* with a combination therapy of cranberry juice and *L. johnsonii La1* probiotics.[35]

More Antibacterial Power of Probiotics

We've created a serious situation in which our perceived best antibiotic drugs are not working against some bacteria, including on serious infectious diseases like MRSA. And it often strikes when people are most vulnerable, such as in hospitals when they are admitted for other health issues. The media have been extensively reporting on the seriousness of the situation and that antibiotic drugs are no longer working against MRSA. But I haven't seen a single media report that showcases a natural option that may work in such cases. Although the research on probiotics in the treatment of antibiotic-resistant infectious diseases like MRSA is

It's All in the Strain—H. Pylori (Part 2)

One thing that really stands out in the research on *H. pylori* infections is the variation in results among different strains of probiotics and the importance of choosing the strains that have demonstrated effectiveness. The probiotic strains *L. johnsonii La1*, *L. reuteri*, and *Saccharomyces boulardii* have, at the time of writing this book, shown the greatest effectiveness against *H. pylori*, whereas *L. paracasei*, *L. acidophilus LB*, *L. GC*, *B. animalis*, and *L. gasseri OLL2716* have been only minimally effective or not effective at all.[36] Although some detractors from the studies might declare after reading one of the studies that probiotics don't work against *H. pylori*, a more accurate assessment would consider that the probiotic strain used makes all the difference. When it comes to using probiotics against *H. pylori*, there is no one-size-fits-all remedy.

As with all research on probiotics, further research is needed to help us use them most effectively, but if you're looking to eradicate an *H. pylori* infection, consider adding *L. johnsonii La1*, *L. reuteri*, and *S. boulardii* to your treatment plan.

in its infancy, it exists and has somehow not caught the attention of mainstream journalists.

A study published in the *International Journal of Antimicrobial Agents* found that probiotics can play a role in the prevention and treatment of MRSA infections. Scientists at Bio-Assistance in Montreal, Canada, found that many strains exhibited antibacterial activity against the superbug that causes the disease.

Probiotics are not just proving effective for the prevention and treatment of highly aggressive infectious diseases like MRSA; they are also demonstrating effectiveness against *Clostridium difficile* infections. *C. difficile* "has surpassed methicillin-resistant

It's All in the Strains—MRSA and S. *Aureus* Infections

Probiotics are showing great promise against MRSA and *S. aureus* infections, which is a great thing now that many of our antibiotics are no longer working against these conditions.

In studies the most active strains against MRSA include *L. reuteri, L. rhamnosus GG, Propionibacterium freudenreichii, P. acnes, L. paracasei, L. acidophilus, L. casei, L. plantarum, L. bulgaricus, L. fermentum,* and *L. lactis.* In animal studies *B. bifidum* showed the greatest efficacy against *Staphylococcus aureus* in vaginal infections, whereas *L. plantarum* had the greatest effect against general *S. aureus* infections and when applied topically for skin wound infections.

Unlike antibiotics, which only ever worked by killing bacteria, scientists found that probiotics worked on *S. aureus* in three ways. First, most of the effective probiotic strains competed with *S. aureus* bacteria for nutrients and attachment and, second, produced acids or antibacterial compounds known as "bacteriocins" to kill the infectious bacteria. Third, *L. acidophilus* inhibited *S. aureus* from producing what is known as a "biofilm," or a coating that protects it and reduces the likelihood of being detected and killed by the immune system. The scientists ultimately concluded that the research "pointed to the feasibility of elimination or reduction of MRSA colonisation with probiotic use."[37]

Additional research published in the *Journal of Medical Microbiology* found that *B. longum* subspecies *longum (ATCC 15707)* and *Bifidobacterium animalis* subspecies *lactis (BCRC 17394)* inhibited the growth of various strains of MRSA.[38] Although there is no guarantee that these probiotic strains will be effective against all MRSA infections, the probiotics are showing greater effectiveness than the antibiotic drug options.

Staphylococcus aureus as the number-one cause of hospital-acquired infections in some areas of the USA," according to research presented in the *International Journal of Infectious Diseases.*[39]

Probiotics Against Viruses—Including the Common Cold

By now you have an understanding of how probiotics work against harmful bacteria, but they also hold great promise in the treatment of viral diseases, including viruses linked to the common cold, cold sores, and AIDS (HIV). The research is still in its infancy regarding HIV, but probiotics are showing that they are not just helpful with bacterial infections and can help our bodies when we're dealing with viral conditions as well.

The Common Cold. Research published in the *European Journal of Nutrition* found that probiotic strains *L. plantarum HEAL 9 (DSM 15312)* and *L. paracasei 8700:2 (DSM 13434)* reduced the risk of contracting the common cold, something that no drug has ever been able to do. The researchers also found that probiotics cut the duration of the common cold by more than two days. The group taking the probiotics also had a reduction in symptoms if they experienced the common cold—three great reasons to take these probiotics.

Respiratory Infections. In a study published in the *Journal of Science and Medicine in Sport*, researchers at the University of Otago, New Zealand, tested the effects of probiotic supplementation on a group of thirty elite Rugby Union players. Although the test group was small, the study showed the effectiveness of probiotics to prevent upper respiratory infections and to reduce the duration of infection in those who became sick.[40]

Other research confirms probiotics' ability to prevent respiratory and ear infections and to aid their healing. According to research published in the *Journal of Applied Microbiology*, scientists discovered that probiotics compete with harmful disease-causing microbes for nutrients, space, and even the ability to attach to their human hosts to infect them. They found that the probiotics thrived at the expense of the infectious microbes, causing the harmful ones to die off and, in the process, reducing lung and ear infections.[41] Now, that's a side effect worth experiencing.

Infants and Children Benefit Too. Probiotics have a safety record that allows them to be used with infants and children. According to a study in the *Journal of Allergy and Clinical Immunology* conducted by the Department of Paediatrics and Adolescent Medicine, Turku University Hospital, in Turku, Finland, researchers found that probiotic supplements reduced the risk of viral respiratory infections in preterm infants. The probiotic-treated infants experienced significantly fewer infections, which led the scientists to conclude that "probiotics might offer a novel and cost-effective means to reduce the risk of rhinovirus infections."[42] That's something most parents will be thrilled about, particularly because there are no pharmaceutical options, and even if there were, the probiotics have demonstrated no negative side effects. Choose a probiotic that has been formulated for infants or children.

Help for the Elderly. Babies and children aren't the only ones who can benefit from the use of probiotics to prevent or treat lung infections. French researchers conducted a large study of 1,072 elderly patients to see whether a yogurt product containing a particular strain of *Lactobacillus casei* would have any impact on the incidence or duration of respiratory infections. They found shortened infection time in common infectious diseases as well as significant reductions in the incidence of upper respiratory tract infections.[43]

Herpes Virus. Most of us have heard of the herpes virus. There are herpes simplex and herpes zoster forms of the virus. The herpes simplex virus presents itself in two main forms: cold sores or genital herpes.[44] Herpes zoster is the virus linked to chickenpox and shingles. Once in the body the herpes virus is always present, but the use of certain remedies can help it to return to a dormant state. The probiotic *Lactobacillus brevis* may help in this regard, as found by scientists at Sapienza University in Italy. *L. brevis* appears to inhibit the virus's ability to multiply. The higher the dose the scientists used, the more antiviral activity *L. brevis* demonstrated.[45] That's not to say that *L. brevis* isn't effective against herpes zoster, merely that this group of scientists only focused their research on herpes simplex. Other research showed that *Lactobacillus plantarum 8A-P3* was effective at inhibiting the herpes simplex virus type 1.[46]

In another study Ukrainian researchers examined the effects of two probiotic strains, *L. plantarum* and *S. salivarius thermophilus*, against viral infections in animals. They found that the probiotics demonstrated effectiveness at killing flu viruses and genital herpes and even at inhibiting the ability of the HIV virus from reproducing.[47] Viruses rely on reproduction to spread throughout the body and for their survival, suggesting that these two strains of probiotics may be helpful in the treatment of flu viruses, genital herpes, and even the management of HIV.

HIV. So how exactly do probiotics work against viruses? In addition to the methods mentioned earlier in this chapter, new research published in the journal *Clinical and Experimental Immunology* studied the effects of two probiotic strains on the immune system's various functions. They found that different strains may work in different ways: one increased the body's means of marking and activating immune system cells known as T cells, whereas another increased the number of killer T cells.[48] Although this type of research that explores the way in which probiotics boost our natural immune system functions is in its infancy, it gives us insight into which strains are demonstrating the best ability to boost immune function and may prove beneficial in treating individuals with compromised immune systems, like those suffering from serious immune-deficiency disorders like human immunodeficiency virus (HIV).

Other research conducted at the Shiraz HIV/AIDS Research Center (SHARC), Department of Bacteriology and Virology, Shiraz University of Medical Sciences, in Shiraz, Iran, found that the probiotic *Lactobacillus rhamnosus* improved the body's ability to manufacture particular immune system cells.[49] These are large cells that engulf dangerous infections and destroy them by "eating" them. They are akin to the body's own Pac-Man against infections. In HIV and AIDs the immune system becomes compromised and demonstrates a reduced effectiveness against the virus causing the disease, making it difficult to treat. The use of this probiotic strain to assist the immune system and its effectiveness holds promise in engaging the immune system to more effectively fight HIV.

Probiotics Assist with Fungal Infections

Our modern lifestyle often leaves women vulnerable to vaginal infections, either of yeast or fungal origin. Many women use antibiotics to treat these infections or harmful chemical-based douches that actually throw off the natural microbial balance in the vagina and can leave women vulnerable to future infections, such as candidiasis or even HIV, as you learned earlier.

Groundbreaking Research on a Devastating Disease

An estimated 33.2 million people are currently suffering from AIDS, the disease caused by HIV, including 1.3 million sufferers of this tragic disease in North America.[50] Most people would agree that AIDS is a devastating disease. And in many cases the medical treatment is also devastating. Although research on the application of probiotics to HIV is in the early stages, it offers promise and hope for those suffering from AIDS or current treatments.

Research shows that an imbalance of microbes in the vagina, known as dysbiosis, is linked to an increased susceptibility for HIV infection and transmission. In other words, an uneven ratio of harmful vaginal bacteria to probiotic bacteria may make women more vulnerable to contracting HIV. This shows that probiotic supplementation may play a role in preventing such serious diseases. Conversely, the research also shows that HIV infections are often characterized by a vaginal microbial imbalance. Researchers suspect that beneficial microbes may protect against HIV in multiple ways: (1) by the direct production of antiviral compounds, (2) by blocking the adhesion and transmission of the virus, and (3) by stimulating the immune response to destroy the virus.[51] Although this research does not suggest that probiotics can kill the HIV virus or cure the disease, it shows promise for the treatment or supplementary treatment of the illness to directly affect the virus, boost the immune system's response against the disease, and reduce some of the many difficult symptoms of such a serious illness. Considering the seriousness of the disease, such a promise is one that its sufferers will likely greet with excitement.

Additional research also found that various probiotics could have a positive influence on those suffering from HIV and AIDs. In a study on 127 HIV-infected children under the age of sixteen, researchers at

Groundbreaking Research on a Devastating Disease (continued)

the Department of Pediatrics and Antiretroviral Therapy (ART) Center at the S.N. Medical College in Agra, India, assessed the effects of probiotic supplementation on the HIV virus. They found that probiotic supplementation showed significant improvement in white blood cells known as CD4.[52] The CD4 count is a reflection of the strength of the immune system to fight viruses and can indicate the stage of HIV/AIDS in a person suffering from the disease. Probiotic supplementation for six months significantly increased the CD4 count, which indicates a stronger immune system. An increase in this number also tends to reflect an improvement in the condition.

People suffering from AIDS are not only vulnerable to the viral disease itself, but because their immune systems are significantly reduced, they are also prone to contracting other infections, such as candidiasis, which you learned about in the last chapter. In a pilot study presented in the journal *Mycopathologia* researchers assessed the effects of probiotic supplementation through ingestion of yogurt as a way to affect the Candida infection. The researchers observed less Candida colonization when the women consumed probiotics.[53] The data they presented is promising, but because it was a small pilot study, more research needs to be done to shine a light on the potential for probiotics to affect Candida infections and the management of serious diseases like HIV.

Probiotics taken in supplement form or used as vaginal suppositories or douches can assist in the regulation of harmful bacteria or yeasts to lessen the risk of infection or treat infections that have already taken hold.

It's All in the Strains—Yeast Infections and Vaginal Health

Researchers at the Lawson Health Research Institute, Canadian Research and Development Center for Probiotics in London, Ontario, Canada, studied a combination of two probiotic strains, *L. rhamnosus GR-1* and *L. fermentum RC-14*, taken orally to determine their ability to restore vaginal microbial balance. The researchers found that the women who supplemented with the Lactobacilli had a significant increase in vaginal Lactobacilli. They also found a significant drop in yeast and a significant reduction in coliform bacteria (such as *E. coli*) for the Lactobacilli-treated women. Thirty-seven percent of women taking the supplement who had vaginal bacterial or yeast infections returned to normal microbe colonization, whereas only 13 percent of the placebo group did. The scientists concluded that this probiotic combination reduces the colonization of pathogenic bacteria and yeast in the vagina and is safe for daily use in healthy women.[54] And as most women can attest, vaginal infections can be a long-standing problem that can sometimes be difficult to treat.

Addressing Microbial Overgrowth Naturally

If you are dealing with an infection—bacterial, viral, fungal, or parasitic—the many probiotics mentioned above may be helpful. Remember to choose the one(s) mentioned for the particular infectious condition you have (for more on this, see Chapter 5). In addition to the many probiotic strains that have proven themselves invaluable against infectious conditions, there are also many great natural remedies that kill Candida and other harmful microbes in the intestines. We incorrectly assume that antibiotics are the only options or that they are superior to natural remedies that kill infectious microbes. Antibiotics only kill bacteria, but an increasing body of research shows that these drugs are no longer effective against many pathogenic bacteria but still kill many beneficial bacteria in the gut, causing a serious imbalance. Additionally, using antibiotics to kill fungal or yeast infections is completely ineffective.

Here are some excellent, all-natural, proven antimicrobials that, along with probiotics, help address an underlying infection that may be having disastrous effects on your health. Keep in mind that it is important to use whichever one(s) you choose on a daily basis until the infection is resolved:

Coconut Oil. Research at Nigeria's University College Hospital found that coconut oil kills close to 100 percent of yeast cells (even drug-resistant species) on contact thanks to its lauric, caprylic, and capric acid content. These ingredients cause the protective outer wall of yeast cells to split apart, making it easier for the immune system to destroy them. Take three tablespoons of extra virgin coconut oil daily to obtain the benefits found in the study.[55]

Dandelion. Recently researchers have added "superbug killer" to the dandelion's impressive health-boosting résumé, having found high antibacterial activity against *E. coli*, *Bacillus subtilis*, and MRSA.[56] In my experience fresh dandelion is an excellent choice when it is harvested from unpolluted and unsprayed areas, away from roadsides. It can be added to fresh juices or sautéed with some garlic and lemon juice. (Choose young dandelion leaves, otherwise it can be quite bitter.) In lieu of using fresh dandelion you can choose an alcohol extract or tea available from most health food stores or your natural health professional.

Garlic. A natural antibiotic, antifungal, and antiviral agent, garlic is a great addition to your diet. Garlic is best known for its sulphur compounds, particularly allicin, which is the main phytonutrient that boosts immunity and acts as a natural antibiotic. Eating a single clove of raw garlic in your daily diet can help diminish the growth of yeast cells. Add raw garlic to previously cooked foods just prior to eating or throw it in a homemade salad dressing. You can also throw some fresh garlic into your favorite soup, stew, chili, stir-fry, meat, or veggie dish. Forget garlic powder, as most of its health benefits are long gone.

Olive Leaf. Olive leaf, like many other natural antibiotics, is also a good antiviral, making it an excellent choice when the nature of the microbe is not completely known. Drs. O. and B. Lee at the Department of Biomedical Science at CHA University in South Korea found that olive leaf extract was potent against various microbes.[57] Additionally, their research showed that olive leaf exhibited free radical–scavenging abilities. Olive leaf is available in juice form, alcohol extract, and capsule. Because every product is different, it is best to follow package instructions.

Oregano Oil. The king of natural antibiotics, study after study proves the effectiveness of oregano oil. If you think natural remedies aren't as potent as drug ones, you might want to rethink that opinion, especially when it comes to oregano oil. Three volumes of research by Paul Belaiche found that oregano oil killed 96 percent of all pneumococcus bacteria and 92 percent of all neisseria, proteus, and staphylococcus bacteria.[58] Some strains of neisseria are responsible for diseases like gonorrhea or meningitis. Proteus is a type of intestinal infection, and staphylococcus is the culprit in some types of food poisoning. Oregano oil eliminated 83 percent of streptococcus and 78 percent of enterococcus, which are linked with strep throat, scarlet fever, rheumatic fever, toxic shock syndrome, cystitis, wound infections, and anorexia.

Of course, like anything, product strength can vary drastically. Some products are actually marjoram and not oregano at all. So choose a reputable brand backed by research. I like North American Herb and Spice Company's blend called P-73, which includes wild, high-potency oregano harvested in harsh conditions. That might not sound like a big deal, but harsh conditions usually spell stronger active ingredients in the plant, as the health-building phytochemicals usually comprise the plant's immune system. Oregano is available in juice form, oil extract, alcohol extract, and capsule. Because every product is different, it is best to follow package instructions.

Most medical professionals have hardly considered using probiotics in preventing or treating infectious diseases, yet the research shows that it warrants a rightful place against these conditions, particularly as our best drugs are losing their effectiveness, causing harmful side effects, and even increasing the virulence of infectious bacteria. Probiotics, however, have many positive side effects, including improving our gut and overall health, reducing our susceptibility to harmful infections, and in treating or managing many serious chronic conditions.

Chapter 4

New Hope for Serious Illnesses

"All these bacteria that coat our skin and live in our intestines, they fend off bad bacteria. They protect us. And you can't even digest your food without the bacteria that are in your gut. They have enzymes and proteins that allow you to metabolize the food you eat."

—Bonnie L. Bassler, molecular biologist and professor, Princeton University

Wayne Addresses His Allergies

Wayne, a tall middle-aged man, came to see me to see whether I might be able to help him with seasonal allergies. He struggled with many pollens and hay fever, which meant he had a constantly runny nose from April to September. He was tired of the reactions and the difficulty breathing due to nasal congestion and sinusitis.

I explained to him that I had read some exciting research using probiotics for allergies. He said, "You mean yogurt?" I shared that there were some probiotics in yogurt but not all the probiotics I

Wayne Addresses His Allergies (continued)

wanted to use with him were found in yogurt. He agreed to take the *S. cerevisiae* and *L. casei* probiotic supplement, which contained other health-boosting probiotics as well. I explained that these probiotics had shown promise in study participants who had allergies, sinusitis, and nasal congestion, so I thought they might help him too.

I also explained that I wanted him to avoid all dairy products and as much sugar as possible for thirty days. To help address his immediate symptoms while the probiotics went to work at healing at a deeper level, I gave him an alcohol extract, known as a tincture, of the herb nettles, which I use with many people with allergies.

Wayne followed my advice to the letter, to my amazement. He came back a month later and told me he was astounded. He said he thought I might help him, but he didn't expect all of his allergies and symptoms to have disappeared in that time. He asked me whether the natural remedies I gave him worked like the drugs for allergies—whether they would stop working as soon as they are discontinued. I explained that they didn't work that way. The probiotics work to restore beneficial bacteria that would naturally be present in his body but that must have become out of balance. I informed him that he may want to continue taking them for a while to ensure his body has the strains from which he seemed to benefit. I explained that he could give his body a boost every February or March so he was in great shape for spring and to use the probiotics and nettles if he started to feel like the allergies were coming back.

Wayne was so thrilled he could return to the outdoor activities he loved so much. Allergies were no longer reducing his quality of life and preventing him from doing the things he loved.

Probiotic-rich foods and supplements have a rightful place at the forefront of healing many health conditions and diseases, from AIDs to depression, brain disease to cancer, and so much more. They are proving themselves useful within the treatment plans of dozens of illnesses and may even prevent many health concerns, especially as part of an overall healthy diet and lifestyle.

Increasing amounts of research show that various strains of Lactobacilli and Bifidobacteria go well beyond the gut to transform the health of our body. As you learned in the last chapter, they have the ability to destroy harmful bacteria, yeasts, fungi, and viruses. They also have been shown to lower the levels of certain immune system chemicals known as cytokines, both in the gut as well as in the blood that feeds the entire body. That's great news, because large amounts of research have linked inflammation as the common denominator behind many serious health conditions, including arthritis, cancer, heart disease, and many other health concerns. Even mood disorders like depression are increasingly being linked to underlying inflammation.[1] Additional research in the journal *Gut Microbes* found that probiotics can reduce inflammation, offering hope for the many serious conditions linked to inflammation and the millions of people suffering from them.

The Inflammation Connection

Arthritis has always been linked to inflammation in the joints, but it hasn't always been clear that dietary and lifestyle changes could postpone the onset of the disease, alleviate pain, and even reduce or eliminate the underlying inflammation linked to the condition.[2]

Clinical research links inflammation to heart disease, ranging from coronary artery disease to congestive heart failure. We now understand that the body uses cholesterol and other fatty deposits to repair damage inflammation causes within the arteries.[3] In studies chronic inflammation in the body has even been shown to contribute to the growth of cancer cells and tumors.[4]

Many other health conditions have been linked to inflammation, including but not limited to ADD/ADHD, Alzheimer's disease, dental issues, diabetes, migraines, obesity, peripheral neuropathy, thyroid conditions, and stroke.[5]

Most medical treatments of these conditions involve addressing symptoms of the diseases but rarely address the underlying inflammation that is causing the problems. Although addressing the symptoms may be important to the sufferer of the disease, it doesn't help slow the progression or reverse the condition. It is important to tackle the inflammation. Inflammatory cytokines are released into the blood or tissues as part of the body's attempt to heal the disease but are destructive to healthy cells. When inflammation becomes chronic, inflammatory cytokines can wear down cartilage and bodily tissues, leading to further inflammation in the body.

Getting cytokines under control is a key factor in restoring health and preventing or managing inflammatory conditions. Because the majority of inflammatory conditions start in the gut, probiotics play a key role in addressing the inflammation that is underlying many health concerns.[6] Before we discuss the use of probiotics to address the inflammation and several inflammation-linked conditions, let's first explore how inflammation begins in the gut.

As you may recall from our discussions about the gut in Chapter 2, the gut has a semipermeable lining. Many factors affect the degree to which it is permeable, but it also fluctuates in response to various chemical reactions in our body. For example, when you have an argument your adrenal glands pump out the stress hormone cortisol, or when you stay up late to work or party your thyroid levels fluctuate. These hormones cause the intestinal lining to become more permeable fairly quickly.[7]

Additionally, any time beneficial bacteria are reduced in the gut as a result of antibiotic or other medication use, stress, a high-sugar diet, and many other factors, it can set the stage for the immune system to "sound the alarm" and increase the production of immune compounds like cytokines, resulting in increased inflammation and intestinal permeability, or "leaky gut syndrome." The more permeable or "leaky" the gut is, the more that incompletely digested food, toxins, harmful bacteria, viruses, and fungi have access to the bloodstream, where they may cause systemic damage.

If the intestinal lining becomes repeatedly damaged due to ongoing or recurring leaky gut syndrome, the damaged microvilli lose their ability to function properly. They become ineffective at processing and using nutrients we eat that are essential to digestion and our overall health. Digestion becomes further impaired, and we lose the ability to absorb other nutrients our body needs for maintenance and tissue and organ repair. You may become more susceptible to immune system attacks on the substances that permeate into the blood, such as the undigested food and toxins. Your body initiates attacks on these "foreign invaders" by responding with inflammation, allergic reactions, and other symptoms we link to other diseases.[8]

It may not sound that serious, but over time this inflammatory response can lead to serious diseases as your immune system becomes overburdened and the inflammatory triggers continue almost incessantly, damaging your nerves, connective tissues, muscles, joints, and other organs. Although not all of the conditions below are linked to inflammation, most are. The common denominator for all of the conditions below is the fact that probiotics are demonstrating their effectiveness for prevention and/or treatment.

Allergies and Allergy-Related Conditions

Although probiotics may seem unlikely remedies for allergy treatment, research shows that some beneficial bacteria can reduce allergy symptoms and even prevent allergic conditions altogether if they are taken early enough in a person's development. Not all probiotics seem to have the anti-allergic effect, but the right ones can heal the intestinal walls and reduce underlying inflammation in the gut, and that can spell greater healing throughout the body.

And this miracle starts before birth! Research in the *Journal of Allergy and Clinical Immunology* found that probiotic consumption by the mother during pregnancy and in the infant's milk reduced the risk of eczema, which is often linked to allergies. The early probiotic consumption also reduced the incidence of another allergic condition called rhinoconjunctivitis in children. Allergic rhinoconjunctivitis (ARC), an inflammatory disorder of the nose, sinuses, and eyes, is the most common allergic disease. In the last four decades it has dramatically increased in prevalence in industrialized and developing nations. It is estimated to affect up to 40 percent of the population of all countries, ethnic groups, and ages, including infants and children. The symptoms usually involve itchy nose, sneezing, watery mucus, nasal congestion or blockage, and itching or burning eyes, tearing, and redness.[9] Because it is frequently associated with asthma and sinus and ear problems, it can impair quality of life.

Consuming probiotics during fetal development and infancy may be helpful in reducing the incidence of allergies, but probiotics have also been found to help with allergy symptoms later in life as well. According to scientists at the Osaka University School of Medicine, the probiotic *Lactobacillus casei* (*L. casei*) delays the occurrence of allergic symptoms.[10] This probiotic also demonstrated effectiveness at reducing sinusitis and nasal congestion linked to allergies.

Other studies demonstrate the effectiveness of the probiotic yeast known as *Saccharomyces cerevisiae*, which has been shown to have an anti-inflammatory effect on the mucous membranes. Another study also showed that the same yeast reduced congestion and runny noses.[11]

Anxiety and Depression

We live in an incredibly stressful, hectic world, and unfortunately many of us have created lives that are neither healthy nor sustainable. It is not surprising that anxiety disorders are the most common forms of mental illness affecting Americans. According to the Anxiety and Depression Association of America, 40 million American over the age of eighteen suffer from a form of anxiety.[12] That is over 18 percent of the population!

There are numerous reasons why people develop anxiety disorders, but the vast majority can be attributed to one or more of the following factors: genetics, brain health, and/or lifestyle or life events and traumas.

If you're thinking of emotional health, you probably never consider what happens in your gut as a factor, but it is. You might consider work stress, home stress, and family stress, but it is doubtful that you'd think of your gut. However, chronic gastrointestinal disorders are now being linked to altered behavior and higher rates of anxiety and, in particular, depression.[13] The gastrointestinal link to these conditions may shed light on new approaches to treating chronic anxiety and depression.[14] In animal studies conducted at the Department of Medicine at McMaster University, Hamilton, Ontario, Canada, the probiotic *Bifido-bacterium longum* eliminated anxiety and normalized behavior. Although the probiotic didn't eliminate inflammation in the gastrointestinal tract, it instead reduced the excitability of the nerves in the gut that connect through the vagus nerve to the central nervous system and, in doing so, eliminated anxiety.[15]

Although the Canadian scientist did not find an effect on inflammation in the gut, Hungarian scientists did. Hungarian scientists found that intestinal inflammation is one of the factors involved in depression and that treating the inflammation with probiotics along with vitamins B and D and omega-3 fatty acids reduced depressive symptoms.[16]

French researchers have also assessed the role of probiotics— in this instance, *Lactobacillus helveticus R0052* and *Bifidobac-terium longum R0175*—on mood and psychological distress to determine whether these probiotics could have an antianxiety effect. They found that the healthy study participants experienced reduced psychological stress, depression, anger-hostility, and anxiety as well as improved problem-solving skills when taking the probiotics for thirty days.[17]

Obviously, more research needs to be completed to gain a better understanding of the use of probiotics in the treatment of anxiety disorders and depression. Although this research is happening, including these proven strains of probiotics within a larger natural approach to treating depression and anxiety may be helpful for people suffering from these psychological disorders. Of course, probiotics are not replacements for prescribed medications.

Arthritis

....

Anyone who has experienced the debilitating pain and inflammation of arthritis will tell you how much these symptoms can rob a person of the joy of living, from the pleasure of pursuing a beloved hobby to the satisfaction of enjoying a favorite sport. Arthritis pain can interfere with the ability to perform even the simplest of tasks and often prevents sufferers from getting that much-needed, restorative good night's sleep that could help silence an overactive immune system and heal joints.

According to the Centers for Disease Control and Prevention (CDC), an estimated 50 million adults in the United States have been diagnosed with arthritis, which includes various forms of the disease, including rheumatoid arthritis (RA), gout, lupus, and fibromyalgia. Although many categorize arthritis as an "older person's disease," this is a myth. The CDC estimates that 294,000 children under eighteen have been diagnosed with some form of arthritic or rheumatic condition. Considering the vast and growing number of people suffering from this debilitating disease, any natural medicine that offers hope and relief is welcome.

Although drugs may temporarily relieve some of the pain, the flip side is potentially serious: the list of side effects can be worse than the disease itself, particularly when it comes to drugs like Vioxx and Celebrex—both drugs have serious side effects.

Probiotics may offer hope in improving joint function for people suffering from rheumatoid arthritis. In a study of thirty rheumatoid arthritis sufferers published in the journal *Medical Science Monitor*, scientists at the University of Western Ontario, Canada, noted joint function improvement in those who took the probiotics *Lactobacillus rhamnosus* and *Lactobacillus reuteri* compared to those given placebos.[18] Although the researchers could not offer an explanation as to why the probiotics improved joint function, because there are no harmful effects of supplementing with *L. rhamnosus* and *L. reuteri* and doing so may actually offer other health benefits, arthritis sufferers may benefit by adding a probiotic supplement with these strains to their treatment regime.

Other research links gut bacteria and the resulting inflammation to rheumatoid arthritis, which may account for the joint function improvement seen in the above study. Researchers at the New York University School of Medicine linked the prevalence of the harmful intestinal bacteria *Prevotella copri* to the onset of rheumatoid arthritis, which may set off an inflammatory response that begins in the gut—and may initiate rheumatoid arthritis.[19] Additionally, the researchers also found that high levels of *P. copri* resulted in fewer beneficial gut bacteria in people suffering from rheumatoid arthritis, suggesting a gut flora imbalance affecting people with the condition.

If *P. copri* infections are linked to the onset of rheumatoid arthritis and the gut flora imbalance, perhaps supplementing with beneficial probiotics that help to restore gut flora balance will also reduce *P. copri* infections as well. As we discussed earlier, researchers have observed joint health improvements with the addition of *L. rhamnosus* and *L. reuteri*, so only time and additional research will tell if these beneficial bacteria can alter the course of this debilitating disease.

Brain Disease

Many brain disorders fall into the categories of developmental, psychiatric, or neurodegenerative diseases. When we think of brain diseases, Alzheimer's disease, dementia, Lou Gehrig's disease, and Parkinson's disease come to mind. Although the treatment for these conditions tends to be complex, new research suggests that probiotics may warrant a place in the treatment of these brain conditions.

The research into using probiotics for brain health is still fairly recent, but the promise and wide-reaching implications it may hold is exciting, particularly because the incidence of brain disease is on the rise. At the current rate of growth scientists predict that brain disease will outnumber heart disease and cancer combined by the year 2022.[20] Although many people incorrectly think that brain diseases are inevitable genetic "time-bombs" that will affect them if a member of their family was afflicted with one, more and more research into natural medicines like probiotics is showing that there are diet and lifestyle changes people can make to prevent their development.

Probiotics can function as antioxidants in the body, which is not only great for reducing the effects of aging (see page 101), but it is especially good news for sufferers of brain diseases. The brain is particularly vulnerable to free radical damage, especially the 60 percent of our brain that is made up of fat. Probiotics may help to protect the fatty parts of our brain from damage, and this, in turn, may help us prevent brain diseases like Alzheimer's disease, Parkinson's disease, Lou Gehrig's disease, dementia, or others.

Swedish researchers found that *Lactobacillus plantarum* resulted in a 37 percent reduction of the chemicals linked to free radical damage that are elevated in many brain and nerve disorders.[21] Free radical damage has been linked to brain and nerve diseases, making their research particularly welcome for those suffering from brain diseases.[22]

Additionally, new research at UCLA found that consuming certain probiotics could actually produce many brain health benefits, including with sensory and emotional processing. The use of probiotics as a potential treatment for brain disease is still in its infancy, but considering affordability, availability, the lack of side effects, as well as the many other health benefits of using them, it seems a natural fit within a larger treatment plan for brain diseases.

Cancer and Chemotherapy Side Effects

According to the National Cancer Institute, almost 41 percent of men and women will be diagnosed with some form of cancer at some point in their lifetime.[23] This alarming reality is all the more disturbing when we realize how much of this cancer risk can be avoided.

It may surprise you to know that everyone has cancer cells in their body. When we are healthy, our body naturally seeks out these cells and destroys them before they can proliferate and form tumors. When we are exposed to high levels of toxins in our food, air, water, and soil, however, our bodies can be weakened and less capable of fighting off cancer growth.

The key risk factors for cancer include the usual bad habits like drinking, smoking, and illicit drug use. Age is also a risk factor, as most cancers are diagnosed in people over the age of forty-five. This may be linked to a lifetime of poor dietary and lifestyle choices, but it does not preclude young people from getting cancer as well. Cancer is frequently linked to genetics, but most cancer experts give as much credence to lifestyle choices and diet as they do to shared DNA. Cancer rates are also higher in highly industrialized countries like the United States and Canada; it is also more prevalent among low-income and less educated populations.

The research into the use of probiotics in the treatment of cancer or the side effects of chemotherapy and radiation treatment is still in the early stages, but some of it warrants serious consideration.

Probiotics offer healing potential in the prevention and possible treatment of colon cancer. Research at the International University of Health and Welfare Hospital, Japan, found that probiotic supplementation improved the bowels of people suffering from colon cancer.[24]

Probiotics also help reduce the incidence and severity of side effects resulting from chemotherapy and radiation. Scientists at the University of Alberta, Canada, found that probiotic supplementation may reduce the GI complications linked to chemotherapy. Because GI complications can compromise the efficacy of chemotherapy, probiotic supplementation may play a role in improving the effectiveness of chemotherapy treatments in people suffering from cancer. Additional research at St. Peter's University Hospital in New Brunswick, Canada, found that probiotics also aided in preventing diarrhea caused by radiation therapy.

From the research we now know that probiotics can play a role as anticancer agents, at least with colon cancer, as well as potentially improving the efficacy of chemotherapy and reducing the ill effects of radiation therapy in treating cancer. Other research on smokers, who are definitely at a disadvantage when it comes to cancer, found that probiotic supplementation exerted a beneficial effect on the immune system. According to research in the *British Journal of Nutrition*, daily intake of the probiotic *Lactobacillus casei Shirota* increased natural killer cell activity in smokers. That might sound like a bad thing, but natural killer cells are one of the immune system's weapons against cancer and other illnesses, so increasing their numbers, particularly in smokers who tend to have lower levels of these immune compounds, may help protect them against cancer.[25]

Diabetes

....

D iabetes is a severe chronic health condition characterized by elevated blood sugar levels. If these levels become too high, they are toxic to the person's organs, including the brain. People with diabetes experience one of two main problems when it comes to handling sugar. They may have a deficiency of insulin, the hormone used to process sugar. Alternatively, the person's cells may be resistant to insulin, causing the blood sugar to be unable to enter the cells.

Over 8 percent of Americans—about 25 million children and adults—have diabetes. That includes type 1 or juvenile diabetes, in which the individual has severe insulin deficiencies. It also includes type 2 diabetes, which often strikes adults and can be linked to a diet heavy in refined carbohydrates and sugars, a sedentary lifestyle, and carrying excess weight. It also includes gestational diabetes that can occur in pregnant women due to hormonal imbalances. The latter is usually temporary but important to address for the health of both the mother and the fetus.

Although not a lot of research has specifically been conducted for the use of probiotics in the treatment of diabetes, probiotics have been found to improve the energy balance of the body while also improving its ability to use glucose (sugar) for energy.[26] The ability to turn glucose into energy is impaired in people with diabetes, so this research shows promise as a possible treatment or adjunct treatment for the disease.

Research on people with diabetes aged thirty-five to seventy tested the effects of a probiotic supplement containing *Lactobacillus acidophilus, L. casei, L. rhamnosus, L. bulgaricus, Bifidobacterium breve, B. longum,* and *Streptococcus thermophilus* along with fructooligosaccharides (FOS). The researchers found that the probiotic supplementation resulted in a decrease in C-reactive protein levels, a marker for inflammation, and also prevented a rise in fasting blood sugar levels. Both of these markers indicate improvements in the status of the condition.[27]

Additionally, subclinical inflammation and increased permeability of the gut (recall our discussion about "leaky gut syndrome") have been linked to diabetes.[28] Researchers at the University College Roosevelt in the Netherlands concluded that "probiotics may lead to a novel way to control and even prevent diabetes in general."[29] More research will give greater clues into the ways we can control or prevent diabetes, but probiotics are definitely standing out as treatment possibilities.

Digestive Disorders

Probiotics truly shine in the treatment of digestive disorders, including celiac disease, colitis, Crohn's disease, and irritable bowel syndrome.

Celiac Disease

Celiac disease is a serious food allergy disorder that is triggered by the gluten and gliadin found in many grains such as wheat, oats, barley, and rye as well as foods containing them. Because wheat flour is used as a thickening agent, gluten is found in virtually all prepared, processed, and packaged food, making avoidance of this ingredient very difficult.

Although investigation into the probiotic-based treatment of celiac disease is still in its infancy, new research holds great promise. In celiac disease the small fingerlike protrusions from the walls of the intestines, called villi, are damaged, resulting in misshapen, blunt protrusions. In one study Scandinavian scientists found that the probiotic *L. casei* completely restored villus blunting in the animals they studied.[30] Their preliminary research may offer hope to the many celiac sufferers if the results are similar in humans. It is too soon to know if *L. casei* can reverse this condition in humans, but considering that *L. casei* has only been linked to beneficial health effects it may be worth the supplementation with a guaranteed gluten-free product rich in this probiotic strain.

Colitis

Colitis is a digestive disorder in which the intestinal lining becomes inflamed. Sufferers of this disease typically experience painful inflammation in the colon.[31] Some evidence suggests that it may be linked to a *C. difficile* infection. You may recall from our earlier discussions that *Clostridium difficile* can cause diarrhea, intestinal inflammation, or worse. Scientists at the Department of Medicine at the University of British Columbia, Canada, found that when antibiotics alone failed to address *C. difficile* infection, probiotics along with the antibiotic drugs proved to be an effective treatment of diarrhea linked to *C. difficile* infection in people with colitis.[32] Although extended antibiotic use may not be advisable, in this case it worked along with the probiotics to address the underlying infection linked to the disease.

A study of intestinal microbial diversity in the *Italian Journal of Pediatrics* concluded that "vast potential exists for manipulating the gut microbiota for therapeutic effect, such as use of probiotics" for various bowel conditions, including ulcerative colitis, inflammatory bowel disease (IBD), and Crohn's disease.[33]

Irritable Bowel Syndrome (IBS)

A common disorder, irritable bowel syndrome (IBS), is a collection of symptoms that affects the large intestine, also known as the colon, or bowels—hence the name. Some of the symptoms include cramping, abdominal pain, bloating, gas, diarrhea, and constipation, or alternating diarrhea and constipation.[34] Like other diseases labeled "syndromes," IBS has no known cause. Although there is no single cause attributed to this uncomfortable condition, that doesn't mean there are no known likely causes, some of which may include hidden food sensitivities, erratic eating habits, or imbalances in the flora of the large intestines.

As you learned earlier, dysbiosis is an abnormal ratio of beneficial to harmful bacteria or microbes in the bowels in favor of the harmful bacteria. Because people with IBS typically have imbalances of flora in the large intestines, it is difficult to know with any certainty whether these imbalances preceded the disorder or are a result of the disorder. In other words, is the imbalance a cause or effect of the condition? I believe that it can be both but that when the harmful microbes outnumber the beneficial ones, the imbalance can leave people susceptible to health problems, including IBS and many others, even seemingly unrelated conditions.

Although IBS can be uncomfortable for sufferers, according to medical authorities it does not cause inflammation or increase the risk of colorectal cancer or other diseases of the colon. It is frequently manageable through dietary and lifestyle changes and stress management.[35]

In my experience as a nutritionist and natural health professional, I've found that one of the best ways to manage IBS is to eliminate common food culprits like dairy products, sugary foods (containing natural or synthetic sweeteners), and all fast foods.

At the same time, gradually—and I stress this point for IBS sufferers!—introduce probiotic supplements and probiotic-rich fermented foods into the diet to address the gut flora dysbiosis, which in turn usually helps improve the symptoms of the condition.

A growing body of evidence shows that a disturbance of the flora in the gut may contribute to IBS and its symptoms.[36] Adding probiotics may also reduce the likelihood for food allergies (see the section on allergies on page 84) and the possible damage from gluten in people who are genetically predisposed to a gluten allergy (see the section on celiac disease on page 93). I mention these conditions here because they can also be factors for IBS. Additionally, research also supports the use of probiotic therapy as a way to address the overall condition of irritable bowel syndrome, although some strains of probiotics are more effective than others.

Resolving Other Digestive Problems

The first six months of an infant's life can be difficult for the baby and parents alike. These months are often replete with colic, constipation, reflux, and other GI disorders. Scientists at several universities and hospitals specializing in pediatrics joined together in an effort to study the possible use of probiotics for infants suffering from GI disorders. They found that infants taking the probiotics had improvements in colic, reduced daily amount of time spent crying, and a reduced incidence of constipation—all of which I am sure pleased both the babies and their parents.[37]

In study after study probiotics are demonstrating their capabilities as the darlings of GI therapies. From diverticular disease to traveler's diarrhea and antibiotic-related side effects, probiotics stand out as the therapy of choice.

It's All in the Strains—Irritable Bowel Syndrome

When it comes to irritable bowel syndrome, the strain makes all the difference. In some studies certain strains of probiotics have been extremely effective.

Research conducted at the Department of Medicine at the University of Manchester, England, confirms that *Bifidobacterium infantis 35624* is particularly effective for the condition. The scientists found that probiotics helped IBS sufferers experience less abdominal pain, bloating, bowel dysfunction, straining, and gas by the end of the four-week study.[38]

When exploring the research on probiotics for the treatment of IBS, it quickly becomes obvious that strain matters. Some strains show no effectiveness on the condition at all, whereas others, like the one mentioned above, are impressive in their results. But what happens when many strains are combined? That's the question researchers at the Clinical Enteric Neuroscience Translational and Epidemiological Research (CENTER) Group at the Mayo Clinic College of Medicine asked. To answer the question, they studied a combination of eight strains of probiotics combined under the product name VSL#3 and followed forty-eight patients with IBS, some of whom took the probiotic combination while others took a placebo. They found that combining the probiotics reduced gas and diarrhea but had no effect on other IBS symptoms. VSL#3 includes *B. breve, B. longum, B. infantis, L. acidophilus, L. plantarum, L. paracasei, L. bulgaricus,* and *S. thermophilus.*[39]

South Korean researchers found that another combination of probiotics, which included *L. acidophilus, L. plantarum, L. rhamnosus, B. breve, B. lactis, B. longum,* and *S. thermophilus,* had a significant reduction in overall IBS symptoms and, specifically, reduced diarrhea in those studied.[40] You'll notice that some of the strains are similar to the combination used in the Mayo Clinic study, but others are different. Because both formulations showed effectiveness for IBS, clearly there are numerous ones that work.

Another study of IBS patients administered *L. acidophilus-SDC 2012* and *2013*. The scientists found that those taking the two strains of probiotics had a 23.8 percent reduction in abdominal pain or discomfort.[41]

Adult sufferers of irritable bowel syndrome are not the only ones who can benefit from probiotics. In a study of children with IBS, Italian researchers studied sixty children aged six to sixteen years to assess the effects of supplementing their diet with *Lactobacillus reuteri DSM 17938* for four weeks. The children who received the *L. reuteri* supplement had significantly less pain intensity than those who received the placebo, suggesting that this supplement may be effective for IBS in children.[42]

What does all the research mean for IBS sufferers? It appears that some combinations of probiotics are helpful but that, to date, the greatest relief has come from specific probiotic strains. According to research published in the journal *Therapeutic Advances in Gastroenterology*, *Bifidobacterium infantis 35624* and *Bifidobacterium lactis DN-173–010* have shown the most encouraging results for treating IBS.[43] That doesn't mean that other probiotics won't help address the symptoms and restore bowel flora balance, but it may be beneficial to obtain these particular strains if you can.

Diverticulosis is a disorder in which the colon becomes misshapen and forms pouches. If harmful bacteria and inflammation form in these pouches, the disorder is then referred to as diverticulitis (-itis meaning "inflammation"). Although they are defined as different conditions, most of the time they are found together. A fiber-deficient diet has been linked to this condition. The lack of fiber causes strain on the colon wall, as more effort is required to push food waste through the colon. This can damage weak spots along the length of the colon, causing the pouches to form. However, Italian scientists found that *Lactobacillus casei DG24* was better than a placebo for symptoms linked to diverticular disease.[44]

If you've done much traveling you may already be familiar with the benefits of probiotic supplementation for traveler's diarrhea. Probiotics are often able to provide rapid and effective relief of this troubling problem. Refer to Chapter 6 for more information on traveler's diarrhea.

Heart Disease

Heart disease is a general term used to define a collection of disorders affecting the heart and blood vessels. Coronary heart disease, a build-up of plaque in coronary arteries that compromises the supply of oxygen-rich blood to the heart, is the most common form of heart disease.

According to the CDC, heart disease is the leading cause of death in the United States.[45] An estimated six hundred thousand Americans die annually from heart disease. That is 25 percent of all deaths in the country every year.

The risk factors for heart disease include smoking, high blood pressure, high homocysteine levels, and high LDL cholesterol. The CDC estimates that 50 percent of Americans have at least one of these risk factors. Other factors include a nutrient-deficient, high-fat, high-dairy, high-salt diet; excessive alcohol, coffee, or tea consumption; a sedentary lifestyle; and genetics.

Keep in mind that the best choice for you may be different from someone else experiencing heart disease, depending on your specific markers for the condition. Obviously, some strains are superior at reducing high cholesterol, whereas others are beneficial in quelling the underlying inflammation.

It's All in the Strains—Heart Disease

Few people would consider probiotics as part of a program for people suffering from heart disease, yet new research suggests maybe we should be seriously considering it.

Quadrant Nutrition, LLC, in Hendersonville, North Carolina, studied the effects of various probiotics or probiotics combined with prebiotics on the markers for heart disease. They found that certain probiotic strains, strain combinations, or probiotics and prebiotic combinations were effective at lowering "bad cholesterol" levels and reducing inflammation. They discovered that the probiotic-only formulations that included *Lactobacillus reuteri NCIMB 30242*, *Enterococcus faecium*, and the combination of *Lactobacillus acidophilus La5* and *Bifidobacterium lactis Bb12* were beneficial to heart health. They also identified that the probiotic and prebiotic combinations of *L. acidophilus CHO-220* plus inulin as well as *L. acidophilus* plus FOS decreased LDL ("bad") cholesterol. The researchers also found that these probiotic strains and probiotic/prebiotic combinations were helpful in reducing inflammation.[46]

Additional research supports the use of another probiotic strain in treating heart disease. Researchers found that *Lactobacillus plantarum TN8* reduced cytokines, those inflammation-causing compounds we discussed earlier, as well as triglycerides, cholesterol levels, and body weight.[47] The scientists who conducted the study concluded that this probiotic strain "exhibited a number of attractive properties that might open new promising opportunities for the improvement of various (health) parameters related to animal health performance and the avoidance of antibiotics and drugs."

The probiotic strain *Enterococcus faecium M-74* has also been found to reduce high cholesterol levels.[48]

The strain *Lactobacillus reuteri NCIMB 30242* has been found to help drop C-reactive protein levels.[49] C-reactive protein (known as

CRP) is produced by the liver. The level of CRP rises when there is inflammation throughout the body, which in turn can be linked to heart disease.[50]

When it comes to using probiotics for treating and preventing heart disease, clearly the strain you choose is an important factor.

Infant Nutrition

It's never too early to start good nutrition. The addition of probiotics through the mother's diet for nursing children may help to prevent health problems later in life. Researchers have found that the early addition of probiotics, including *Lactobacillus rhamnosus GG, L. casei Shirota, Bifidobacterium animalis, Bb-12, L. johnsonii La1, B. lactis DR10,* and *S. cerevisiae boulardii,* can activate the child's immune system and help prevent immune system disorders in childhood.

Pregnant and nursing women can also improve their baby's health through probiotic supplementation. Finnish researchers found that women who supplemented with *L. rhamnosus* and *Bifidobacterium lactis* provided breast milk of higher nutritional quality to their nursing children than women who did not supplement with the probiotics.[51]

Aging

Infancy isn't the only time in life when probiotics are beneficial. Probiotic supplementation may also be beneficial during the later years.

Antioxidants are the key protectors of the body's cells because they actively protect cells against free radical damage. Free radicals are charged molecules that result from normal metabolic processes, harmful toxins, or other substances that are responsible for damage to tissues and the resulting disease or signs of aging such as wrinkling, joint damage, and so forth. They cause damage to otherwise healthy tissue in the body, depending on where they are found. Free radicals have been linked to virtually all diseases and the aging process because they essentially speed up aging and disease. When we normally talk about antioxidants we are discussing some of the main nutrients that have demonstrated significant antioxidant activity, such as vitamins A, C, and E; selenium; and alpha lipoic acid. However, new research shows that some probiotics also act as important antioxidants in the body. They have been shown to protect against free radical damage and against damage to the fatty components of cells in particular.[52] Lactobacilli and Bifidobacteria seem to particularly demonstrate the ability to act as antioxidants in the body. Probiotics can actually seem to slow the aging process.

It seems like a natural fit to use probiotics to fight off harmful infections. Then we can let the bugs battle it out. Yet few people would consider probiotics as part of an antiaging regime or a program to heal from depression, brain disease, or heart disease. But the research shows these applications aren't so outlandish at all. The promise of probiotics seems unending.

Chapter 5

How to Select Probiotic Supplements

"Bacteria are not germs but the germinators—and fabric—of all life on earth. In declaring war on them we declared war on the underlying living structure of the planet—on all life-forms we can see—on ourselves."

—Stephen Harrod Buhner, *The Lost Language of Plants*

Samantha Experiences Less Depression

Twenty-seven-year-old Samantha came to see me after battling depression for several years. She couldn't remember the exact date it started, but she confessed that she couldn't remember feeling happy in her life. We explored the potential benefits of working with a counselor, which she agreed to do. Then we got to work on her diet and lifestyle to make them better support her emotional needs.

Like many people I've seen with depression, Samantha ate a lot of sugar and refined carbohydrates, which feed harmful bacteria in the intestines and can contribute to blood sugar and hormonal imbalances linked with depression. I ran some saliva hormone tests to get

Samantha Experiences Less Depression (continued)

a clearer picture of her hormone health, which was actually pretty good, so I knew we needed to work on low-grade inflammation and intestinal bacterial imbalances. Because the gut is an integral starting point for both of these concerns, I asked her to follow a gut health diet and lifestyle and to take probiotic supplements.

I explained that there was some exciting research that found probiotics like *B. longum* and *L. helveticus* had lessened depression and anxiety. Although she understood that the research was in its early stages, she was eager to try anything that might help her, particularly something natural with virtually no side effects. Because probiotics alone would likely help but not necessarily address all aspects of the condition, we explored Samantha's diet. I asked her to remove all foods containing additives such as artificial sweeteners and MSG and to significantly cut back on sugar in her diet, as these items have been linked to depression and mood imbalances. I also asked her to eat every two to three hours to avoid blood sugar fluctuations that can aggravate the condition.

In addition to the probiotic supplements and probiotic-rich foods I asked her to take daily, she also started taking 3000mg of fish oil daily. Because so many B-complex vitamins are involved in healthy mood balance, I recommended a 50mg B-complex with two meals each day. Then she added an herbal extract of St. John's Wort (thirty drops three times daily) because multiple studies have found that this powerful herb is effective in reducing mild to moderate depression. Finally, at bedtime she began taking 50mg of 5-HTP, a natural nutritional supplement that has also been found to help with depression.

I asked her to start writing out her feelings in a journal whenever she felt stressed or depressed and to go for a walk during daylight hours (preferably in the morning) every day because both regular exercise and moderate sunlight exposure have been found to be helpful when combating depression.

Samantha followed my plan and returned in a month to report that she felt about 60 percent improved, which I was quite happy with, considering only a month had passed. She agreed to continue the program and report back in another month, at which time she said she felt 90 percent improved. She still felt depressed occasionally, but most of the time she felt happier, as though a fog had lifted around her. She declared that the greatest change had been in her outlook: she now understood that even when she felt depressed, she had tools at her disposal to empower her to feel better.

Most people find the probiotics section of their local health food store daunting. Every company and salesperson claims their product is king and proceeds to tell you why you need twelve strains of probiotics, billions of colony-forming units (CFUs), live cultures, and added *prebiotics*. The discussion on *prebiotics* then leads to the mention of the importance of FOS and inulin and maybe suggestions for other products you should buy too. Much of the information provided tends to be exaggerated or inaccurate, causing endless confusion for consumers and anyone looking to improve their health.

In this chapter I will connect the dots between all the information about probiotics and various health conditions and explain everything you need to know to purchase probiotic supplements. I will outline the difference between *prebiotics* and *probiotics*, different types of cultures, which strains of bacteria you absolutely want, and other information that will help you to select the probiotic supplement that is right for you. I offer suggestions on particular strains you should look for to help combat particular illnesses. I'll help to dispel the confusion and the myths around probiotics and prebiotics and explore consumer tests that examined probiotics in the laboratory to see whether they measured up to their own claims. I'll also tell you how to find out whether your yogurt is all it's cracked up to be and whether it even contains any "live cultures" at all, contrary to what the label might indicate.

Before we delve any further, let's first explore the difference between probiotics and prebiotics because there is a tremendous amount of confusion between the two and whether prebiotics are a necessary addition to your probiotic supplement.

The Pros of Probiotics

As you learned earlier, probiotics are microorganisms that promote health. But let's recap briefly in the context of the difference between probiotics and prebiotics. Probiotics are primarily bacteria as well as the occasional yeast culture that confers health benefits when eaten or taken in supplement form. As you discovered in Chapters 3 and 4, there are many different strains of bacteria that offer an array of health benefits, ranging from boosting immunity and reducing arthritis symptoms to boosting brain health and fighting cancer.

These bacteria are primarily from the Lactobacilli, Bifidobacteria, and, occasionally, from the Saccharomyces (yeast) families (you'll find out more about these in just a bit). These healthy bacteria "crowd out" harmful pathogenic bacteria and yeasts in the intestines, helping to prevent and heal various health concerns mentioned in the previous chapters.

Of course, as you learned in Chapter 2, unheated or unpasteurized fermented foods like yogurt, kimchi, sauerkraut, and others also naturally contain many probiotics, which we'll discuss a bit further later in this chapter. After all, you may be wondering how you can tell whether your yogurt contains live cultures. I'll teach you a simple test you can do at home to help you find out.

Dispelling the Myths About *Prebiotics*

Like us, probiotics need food to survive. *Prebiotics* are the foods that feed probiotics and enable them to populate the intestines. Many food products and supplements come with claims that they contain prebiotics that are necessary for probiotics to work, but that isn't the whole story. In most cases adding prebiotics to packaged foods or supplements isn't necessary unless you eat a poor diet or have extremely weak digestion. And if you eat a poor diet, I hope that by now you've gained the message that it is critical to make changes to improve your diet.

For most people the addition of *prebiotics* to probiotic supplements is really more of a marketing strategy, in my opinion. Although there is some excellent research showing that added prebiotics encourage the growth of probiotics, the truth is that if you're eating a diet high in fiber along with fruit, vegetables, grains, and legumes, you're probably getting all the prebiotics that beneficial bacteria need to thrive inside your gut.

When it comes to probiotic supplements, a small amount of added FOS or inulin (see below for more info on these) may be great, but in others they may waste valuable "real estate" space inside the tiny capsules that is better served with probiotics. Here's why: prebiotics are carbohydrates such as sugars, starches, and fiber and are found in all plant-based foods. Of course, some are better than others. Although research shows that prebiotics fuel probiotics and help them to proliferate, the reality is that most people should be getting prebiotics from their daily diet. Once the probiotics feed on these substances in your gut and proliferate, they'll help improve your gut health and overall health. But you'll have to make a concerted effort to eat more fermented foods or take probiotic supplements to get adequate *probiotics*.

Here are some instances when added prebiotics are helpful:

- You eat a poor diet replete with fast foods.
- You alternate between eating a poor diet and a healthy diet but really don't stick to healthy eating on a daily basis.
- You eat animal protein like burgers, steak, chicken, pork, or other type at almost every meal.
- You have less than one daily bowel movement.
- You have had issues with constipation, diverticulitis (misshapen and inflamed intestines), or diverticulosis (misshapen intestines).
- Your diet tends to go up and down a lot due to traveling or other circumstances.
- You drink fewer than six cups of water daily.
- You don't make an effort to eat a lot of fibrous foods (fewer than thirty-five grams daily).

What About FOS and Inulin?

If you read "contains FOS" or "fructooligosaccharides" on the package of probiotic supplements, keep in mind that "oligosaccharides" are simply sugar molecules and "fructo" simply indicates that these sugars are derived from fruit. Inulin is a type of fiber that is also touted as a popular prebiotic.

Many products indicate that they have "Added *Prebiotics*" or "Contains *Prebiotics*" or "Added FOS" or "Added Inulin" or something like that. In most cases it may actually mean that the product contains sugar, which most people need less of, not more.

Food Sources of *Prebiotics*

There are many great sources of prebiotics in a healthy diet. Some of the best ones include:

asparagus

bananas

burdock

chicory root

dandelions

endive

garlic

Jerusalem artichokes

leeks

onions

radicchio

Eat more of these foods and other foods rich in fiber to give the beneficial bacteria a boost.

So be sure to check the ingredients to see whether there is simply added sugar in the product you've selected. Keep in mind that any ingredient that ends in "-ose," such as fructose, glucose, galactose, and so forth, is another word for sugar.

Probiotics: Meet the Family

There are many different types of bacteria that colonize the body—we've talked about many of them in previous chapters. Here let's focus on some of the main ones. The two main types of bacteria are Lactobacilli and Bifidobacteria. These groups of bacteria, each of which has many species and subspecies, perform vital functions in your body, enabling you to obtain the nutrients you need to build a strong body, detoxify toxic substances that would otherwise harm you, stimulate your immune system to protect you against harmful bacteria and viruses, and keep your intestines healthy and strong to prevent inflammation and disease there or elsewhere in your body.[1]

Some of the species showing the most promise to prevent disease include strains such as *Lactobacillus acidophilus, brevis, casei, plantarum, reuteri,* and *rhamnosus* along with *Bifidobacteria lactis* and *bifiform.* Although these names may sound like a foreign language, you'll soon discover that most of these beneficial bacteria are found in readily available fermented foods and supplements. Many of these medicinal powerhouses float around in the air, just waiting for the opportunity to proliferate on foods and in beverages as well as to share their healing powers with us in exchange for the opportunity to co-exist in our bodies.

Meet the Lactobacilli Family

The most widely known strains of probiotics are members of the Lactobaccilli family. They are primarily found in the small intestines; mucous membranes of the nose, throat, mouth, and genitals; and upper respiratory tract. They are involved in cellular renewal to keep the walls of the intestines healthy. Pregnant women tend to have particularly large colonies of these healthy bacteria, which will then inoculate a newborn so he or she will have the beneficial bacteria needed for health.

You'll notice that the name *Lactobacillus* is often shortened to *L.* when referring to specific strains of bacteria. There are many different strains in the Lactobacilli family, including *L. acidophilus,*

L. brevis, L. bulgaricus, L. casei, L. delbueckii, L. gasseri, L. john-sonii, L. paracasei, L. plantarum, L. reuteri, L. rhamnosus, and *L. salivarius,* all of which produce lactic acid and hydrogen peroxide in the intestines. Hydrogen peroxide has naturally antimicrobial qualities and tends to kill viruses, fungi, and disease-causing bacteria. Lactobacilli also trigger anti-inflammatory proteins produced by white blood cells, which respond to harmful invaders of the immune system to help our bodies fight infection.

Lactobacillus acidophilus is the first strain of probiotic I learned about twenty-five years ago and one of only a handful known by health professionals at that time—and it may be the one you've heard of most. Since then we've discovered many other health-promoting strains in this family.

They convert various types of sugars to lactic acid, which is why they are valuable in food fermentation procedures that preserve food. Some strains of Lactobacilli are found in fermented foods like yogurt, fermented vegetables and sauerkrauts, pickled vegetables, sourdough bread (although they are killed during the baking process), fermented beverages like kombucha (typically green or black tea that has been fermented), and fermented fruit dishes. (For more about these fermentation processes and how to employ them in your kitchen, see Chapter 6.)

Lactobacillus acidophilus—The First Discovered Probiotic

Before many of the other valuable probiotics were known, beneficial bacteria were often called "acidophilus." Now, frequently shortened to *L. acidophilus, Lactobacillus acidophilus* is a strain of bacteria that is commonly found in yogurts with live cultures. It ferments milk sugars, known as lactose, along with many other sugars and carbohydrates. It also helps to break down gluten, a specific type of protein found in wheat, oats, rye, and many other grains.[2] It is important to replenish *L. acidophilus* during and after antibiotic use.

Lactobacillus brevis—The Booster of Anticancer Compounds

L. brevis tends to adhere well to the intestinal walls, which means it assists in "crowding out" harmful disease-causing agents (pathogens). It helps to break down compounds known as polyamines, which have been linked to vaginal infections and intestinal cancer. This strain of bacteria also increases our body's production of anticancer compounds known as interferons.[3]

Lactobacillus bulgaricus—The Cholesterol Normalizer

L. bulgaricus is a close relative of *L. acidophilus*. It has been extensively used in the production of yogurt and cheese. It helps restore normal cholesterol levels and reduces the LDL cholesterol (sometimes referred to as the "bad" cholesterol). Like many of its Lactobacilli family members, it reduces inflammation, which means it may hold promise for serious illnesses, as you discovered in Chapters 3 and 4.[4]

Lactobacillus casei—The Dairy Digester

L. casei helps to break down a compound called casein found in dairy products as well as gluten found in many grains. It helps to regulate immune responses and antagonizes the harmful bacteria *Helicobacter pylori*, which have been linked to many health concerns, including ulcers, and fights *E. coli* bacteria to reduce the likelihood of food poisoning. *L. casei* also helps reduce cytokines, substances in the body that cause inflammation.[5]

Lactobacillus gasseri—The Destroyer of Harmful Bacteria

L. gasseri is present in the human gut and in healthy women's breast milk and vaginas. *L. gasseri* produces compounds that naturally kill harmful bacteria (called bacteriocins), particularly infectious diseases linked to Clostridium, Listeria, and Enterococcus. *Clostridium difficile* (*C. difficile*) can cause diarrhea, intestinal inflammation, and, in severe cases, death.[6] Listeria is a food-borne pathogen that has been linked to meningitis and inflammatory gastrointestinal diseases like gastroenteritis as well as blood poisoning.[7] Enterococcus are bacteria that cause infections typically acquired during a hospital stay and can infect the urinary tract, wounds, or the heart.[8]

Lactobacillus paracasei—The Warrior for Good

L. paracasei has wide-reaching benefits. It contributes to healthy vaginal microbial balance, balances intestinal flora, and even helps reduce nasal and sinus congestion linked to allergies. It is an excellent warrior against pathogenic bacteria like *Clostridium difficile* (*C. difficile*) and *Staphylococcus aureus* (*S. aureus*). *S. aureus* is the culprit behind MRSA that we've been hearing about so much in the news lately. It is one of the pathogenic bacteria that causes infection and no longer responds to antibiotic use.[9] Fortunately, *L. paracasei* can help.

Lactobacillus plantarum—The Restorer of Healthy Intestines

This beneficial bacteria is generally lacking in people eating the Standard American Diet (SAD) but is commonly found in people eating a traditional plant-based diet. It is best known for its ability to reduce inflammation-causing compounds, making it beneficial in the treatment of diseases linked to inflammation such as arthritis, cancer, diabetes, and heart disease. It is helpful to restore healthy intestinal walls and is a warrior against *C. difficile* infection. It is also helpful in treating irritable bowel syndrome.[10]

Lactobacillus reuteri—The Versatile Healer

L. reuteri has demonstrated effectiveness in many different areas of health. It reduces infections and diarrhea linked to infections in infants and children and has shown promise in treating side effects of chemotherapy in adult cancer patients. *L. reuteri* is also one of the most potent probiotics against the *H. pylori* infection that has been linked to ulcers. It is effective against the infection linked to the dental condition periodontitis, which is linked to excessive wear of the teeth and inflammation of the gums. Still other research shows that *L. reuteri* may help reduce inflammation in the body that has been linked to heart disease and other chronic conditions.

Lactobacillus rhamnosus—The Anti-Inflammatory Bacteria

L. rhamnosus may sound more like an Egyptian god, but it warrants this elevated status among bacterial colonies. This member of the Lactobacilli family manufactures enzymes, which are specialized types of proteins. In this case the enzymes are highly anti-inflammatory, causing *L. rhamnosus* to hold great promise in treating inflammatory conditions. It also enhances our natural immunity to disease and is a particularly good warrior against *E. coli* and *C. difficile*. It may also support immune health in infants with allergies.[11]

Lactobacillus salivarius—The Calcium Enhancer

If you're worried about osteoporosis, make friends with *L. salivarius*. This strain of the Lactobacilli family actually enhances the body's absorption of calcium, and this is just one of its many benefits. It is found in healthy intestines and mucus membranes such as the mouth, nose, eyelids, and genitals. It reduces inflammation in the body and even secretes substances that kill harmful microbes.[12] It fights the harmful bacteria *Salmonella typhimurium*, which causes diarrhea and intestinal inflammation.[13]

Meet the Bifidobacteria Family

The Lactobacilli family cannot take all of the credit for helping us stay healthy. The Bifidobacteria family is another powerful family of health-promoting bacteria. They are most commonly found in the mouth, GI tract (especially the large intestines), and vaginal areas. Their function varies from strain to strain, but some of the benefits they confer include vitamin production, destroying cancer-causing compounds, destroying harmful infection-causing microbes, and balancing the immune system.[14]

The name *Bifidobacterium* is often shortened to *B.* when referring to specific strains of bacteria. There are about thirty identified strains of Bifidobacteria so far, with the most common ones being *B. bifidum*, *B. breve*, *B. infantis*, *B. lactis*, and *B. longum*.

There are about seven times as many Bifidobacteria than Lactobacilli present in a healthy adult gut. Newborn babies that have been breastfed tend to have an especially large number of Bifidobacteria, as they receive it through their mother's milk; this helps the baby to prevent harmful infections in childhood and throughout his or her life. Bifidobacteria are strong boosters of the immune system. Some strains of Bifidobacteria are found in yogurt, kefir, fermented vegetables such as sauerkraut, and kombucha.

Bifidobacterium bifidum—The Preventer of Allergies

B. *bifidum* are present in large numbers in the large intestine, or colon as it is often called. However, due to antibiotic use, poor diet, and possibly other factors, their numbers are often reduced. Research shows that B. *bifidum* colonies are reduced in infants suffering from allergies.[15] As a result, restoring this strain of bacteria may be helpful in alleviating allergies. It has been shown to regulate and strengthen the immune system against harmful microbes such as C. *difficile*. It is important to replenish B. *bifidum* during and after antibiotic use.

Bifidobacterium breve—The Destroyer of Infectious Diseases

B. *breve* secrete enzymes that favorably alter intestinal microbes. These enzymes actually kill harmful microbes that are linked to infection and disease, including those linked to Clostridium species such as C. *difficile*.[16] B. *breve* also keep Bacteroides, another group of bacteria, in healthy numbers. Although Bacteroides can be beneficial in the intestines, if their numbers become too high or they migrate beyond the intestines, then they can be responsible for abscesses or other infections.[17] B. *breve* also stimulate the body's ability to produce antibodies, which improve our ability to overcome infectious diseases. B. *breve* is a warrior against infections caused by *Campylobacter jejuni* and rotavirus.

Food Poisoning—and Good Bacteria

Did you know that C. jejuni is the number one cause of food-borne illness in the United States and that rotavirus is the cause of 600,000 to 850,000 deaths annually?[18]

It's true. Fortunately, the probiotic B. breve has been shown to stimulate the body's ability to overcome infectious diseases like C. jejuni and rotavirus. B. breve has been found in studies to be a warrior against infections and a worthwhile addition to your medicine cabinet.

Bifidobacterium infantis—The Baby Health Builder

Based on the name, you can probably guess where this bacteria is primarily located: B. infantis is typically found in the intestines of infants. It is rarely found in adults. It is a strong warrior against one of the harmful strains of bacteria believed to play a causal role in inflammatory bowel disease, *Bacteroides vulgatus*. B. infantis also reduces compounds that cause inflammation and are involved in many inflammation-linked illnesses, ranging from depression to arthritis. Combined with *L. acidophilus*, it helps reduce diarrhea and restores healthy microbial balance in the intestines of infants, particularly when the flora balance is thrown off from antibiotic use.[19]

Bifidobacterium lactis—The Anti-Tumor Superhero

B. lactis is a superhero when it comes to tumors and infections. It secretes a compound that kills harmful microbes and boosts the tumor cell–killing properties of the immune system. It also boosts the immune system cells that fight disease and significantly improves the immune system's ability to cope with cholera and tetanus.[20]

Bifidobacterium longum—The Bacterial GI Joe

B. longum is frequently the dominant strain of Bifidobacteria found in humans. Recall our earlier discussion about the significant amount of variation among bacteria found in one human to another, and you'll have a clear idea why I say "frequently" the dominant strain. As we're discovering with the Human Microbiome Project, bacterial composition is much like fingerprints: no two humans have exactly the same numbers and strains of bacteria. *B. longum* reduces intestinal inflammation and fights *E. coli* bacterial infections. It helps restore a balanced immune response and reduces lung and respiratory inflammation. It also reduces the amount of inflammation found in people with ulcerative colitis.[21]

Other Health-Promoting Bacteria

The Lactobacilli and Bifidobacteria families are not the only beneficial microbes. In addition to these two families, *Streptococcus thermophilus* is another primary probiotic used for boosting health. As time goes on, scientists are likely to discover many other beneficial microbes as well. For now, let's explore *S. thermophilus*.

Streptococcus thermophilus—The Gene Genie

When you read or hear "strep" you probably think of "strep throat" and the bacteria that cause this nasty ailment, but not all strep bacteria are evil. *S. thermophilus*, which is commonly used in yogurt and cheese production, strongly inhibits harmful microbes in food items and in our bodies. It even protects the body against carcinogens and reduces any DNA damage and premalignant lesions they may cause. It helps support healthy GI functions, improves rotavirus-caused diarrhea, and has been linked to remission in ulcerative colitis.[22]

Beneficial Yeasts and Fungi

Beneficial yeasts and fungi are naturally found in our bodies as well. In balanced amounts they promote health. Beneficial yeasts are involved in the fermentation processes of many different foods, including beer, sourdough bread, and wine. Yeasts are naturally present in soil and air; that's how airborne yeasts populate these foods to ferment them. Beneficial yeasts are not related to disease-causing ones such as *Candida albicans* and do not contribute to Candida overgrowth (for more on Candida, see page 26). By comparison, yeasts are much larger than bacteria, although neither is visible to the naked eye. Our knowledge of beneficial yeasts is likely in its infancy, but we do know that *Saccharomyces boulardii* offers many health benefits.

Saccharomyces boulardii—The Anti-Diarrhea Remedy

S. boulardii may sound like a Bollywood superstar but is actually a beneficial yeast. The French microbiologist Henri Boulard observed Indo-Chinese people treating diarrhea resulting from cholera with a fermented lychee and mangosteen tea. When he examined the beverage he found a strain of yeast not previously identified and named it *Saccharomyces boulardii*. He patented the probiotic as an anti-diarrhea drug.[23] *S. boulardii* is effective against diarrhea because it has broad antimicrobial effects against harmful microbes, including *C. difficile*, *E. coli*, *Candida albicans*, and other pathogens found in the GI tract. It also helps Bifidobacteria populations expand.[24]

How Much Should I Take?

Every probiotic product is different, but usually 1 to 10 billion living organisms (or CFUs) is sufficient for most people. Ideally, take probiotics on an empty stomach or twenty minutes before eating and an hour or two after eating. They are best taken first thing in the morning or before bed and can be taken in divided doses throughout the day, if you prefer. Take capsules with some water or juice or mix the powdered form directly into water or juice.

What to Look for in a Probiotic Supplement

Supplement your diet with a high-quality probiotic, preferably one from a reputable company to help ensure that you're getting what you pay for. It may seem confusing because there are so many different possible strains found in the vast array of probiotic supplements in the marketplace. Some contain *Lactobacillus acidophilus* only, whereas others contain many different bacterial strains such as *Streptococcus thermophilus, Propionibacterium freudenreichii, Lactobacillus rhamnosus, Lactobacillus plantarum, Lactobacillus paracasei, Lactobacillus bulgaricus, Lactobacillus acidophilus, Bifidobacterium longum, Bifidobacterium lactis, Bifidobacterium infantis, Bifidobacterium breve,* and *Bifidobacterium bifidum,* and possibly others.

There are literally thousands of different possible strains of bacteria, and not all of them have been proven effective or even safe for inclusion in probiotic supplements. If there is one message I'd like you to take with you about selecting probiotic supplements, it is that a greater variety of strains and higher numbers of bacterial units in a supplement does *not* necessarily make a product superior.

Usually, bacteria are measured in colony-forming units—or CFU for short—and most types will have between 1 and 20 billion CFU. Or the package may just indicate, say, 4 billion per capsule. However, don't be fooled into thinking that choosing a quality probiotic is just a numbers game. A higher number of CFUs does *not* necessarily indicate a superior product.

I wish I could tell you that there is a foolproof way of knowing whether a probiotic supplement is great or lousy. Unfortunately, there isn't a guaranteed way to discern between good- and poor-quality probiotic supplements without trying them, but there are some factors to consider when making your purchase.

Factors to Consider When Purchasing Probiotic Supplements

Reputation of the Company. There are many companies that are simply jumping on the probiotics bandwagon due to the increasing amounts of research and public information about their health benefits. Although there may be nothing wrong with a start-up probiotics manufacturing company, it is best if the company has third-party proof that their product claims are valid. Too many companies are offering the world in their supplements but may not deliver on the claims. In a perfect world companies would report

---

Are There Any Side Effects of Taking Probiotics?

Higher doses of probiotics, however, may cause an increased likelihood of side effects such as bloating, gas, or indigestion. In most cases these effects simply reduce over time as your body becomes accustomed to the addition of probiotic cultures in the diet. Side effects are usually mild.

exactly what is found in their product, but some companies' products do not contain what they claim to contain.

ConsumerLabs.com conducted an extensive study of nineteen probiotic supplements manufactured by different companies in the United States and found that only fourteen products actually provided the amounts of probiotics listed on the labels.[25] (I've listed more information about those products that did not measure up to the claims on page 126.)

Science-Backed Strains. As you've learned, there are many strains of probiotics available, but not all of them are sufficiently researched to warrant inclusion in supplements. A long list of bacterial strains is not necessarily better than well-researched and effective strains proven through research to do what you're hoping they will do for your health. Remember that bacteria compete with each other for nutrition and resources, so dominant strains may simply beat out the strains that are less resilient. The package could say the product has twelve strains, but you might end up with only a few after ingesting them. So you may be paying extra for strains that may not even survive once you've swallowed them. Or you may be paying for strain combinations that are untested through research. Although the "throw everything into the pool" approach may seem like a good idea, it is rarely effective in reality.

Stability. You just discovered that some probiotic strains are unstable and therefore not suited for inclusion in supplement form at all. But that is not the only stability factor to consider. By the time the product has been manufactured, transported, and sits on health food or pharmacy store shelves even before it gets to you, it may no longer contain some of the probiotics reported. Probiotics are measured in CFU, which simply represents the reported number of live bacteria. Product labels usually indicate 1 to 25 billion CFUs of specific probiotic strains. Some companies assert that their product contains 5 billion organisms "at the time of manufacture," which is actually useless information and frankly misleading to consumers. Probiotics can and do die over time, when exposed to heat, or when they are not refrigerated, as well as when they are affected by other factors. Other companies report the number of organisms at the end of the shelf life of the product, which is actually a much more useful number, so opt for products that do this. Companies that report the number of CFUs at the end of the shelf life usually factor in a 50 percent loss of probiotic cultures by the expiration date of the product. In other words, a product that claims to have 10 billion CFUs by the expiration date may actually have many more than that throughout its shelf life. However, as with any type of consumer product, there will always be some products that simply do not contain what they claim to contain. (For more information, check out the box on page 126 regarding products tested by ConsumerLab.com.)

Mixture of Cultures. You may remember our earlier discussion that Lactobacilli are more likely to inoculate the small intestines, whereas Bifidobacteria are more likely to inoculate the large intestines. That needs to be considered when purchasing probiotic supplements. You'll want a mix of both types to ensure that both the small and large intestines are benefiting from the products.

Potency. Most products contain anywhere from 1 to 50 billion active cultures, although the latter rarely occurs in reality, despite what the label might state. Most people benefit from 1 billion CFUs of the specific strains for maintaining general health, but in some cases people may need higher doses.

Should Everyone Use Probiotics?

Although probiotics are beneficial for most people, they may not be right for everyone at every time in life. Probiotics can interact with some medications, and there can be certain circumstances during which time it would be best to reconsider.

Contraindications with Medications. Although some doctors express concern that taking probiotics along with antibiotic treatment can reduce the effectiveness of the antibiotics, I think the concern may be more theoretical than proven. Having said this, if your doctor or pharmacist suggests you avoid probiotics while taking antibiotics, you should follow these instructions.

Additionally, if you are taking medications that are intended to suppress your immune system, such as after a transplant, you may need to avoid taking probiotics. Some medications that decrease the immune system include azathioprine (Imuran), basiliximab (Simulect), cyclosporine (Neoral, Sandimmune), daclizumab (Zenapax), muromonab-CD3 (OKT3, Orthoclone OKT3), mycophenolate (CellCept), tacrolimus (FK506, Prograf), sirolimus (Rapamune), prednisone (Deltasone, Orasone), corticosteroids (glucocorticoids), and others.[26] Check with your doctor or pharmacist.

Other Considerations. Infants should use only a reputable probiotic formulated for infants. Although Lactobacilli are likely safe for most people, including babies and children, not all products may be. Use of probiotics during pregnancy and breastfeeding is probably safe, but many strains of probiotics have not been studied for this application, so their safety may be unknown. Additionally, if you have a weak immune system, you should consult with a physician prior to using probiotics.

Allergies. If you suffer from a gluten, milk, soy, wheat, corn, or other allergy, be sure to check the label to ensure that it doesn't contain traces of these food products. Keep in mind, however, that there can still be minute trace amounts of dairy products, particularly in Lactobacilli strains, as they are usually extracted from dairy products. If you have a severe dairy allergy, check the package and choose products that are guaranteed to be free of dairy products.

Not One Size Fits All. You will need different products at different times in your life. Consider your age and health issues in selecting a probiotic supplement. For example, vaginal infections have been shown in research to respond to *L. rhamnosus GR-1*, whereas *H. pylori* infections have been shown in studies to respond to Bifidobacterium and Saccharomyces strains. Refer to the specific health conditions mentioned in Chapters 3 and 4 to help you when selecting the right strains for your specific health needs. And if a store salesperson tells you that they have a product that works on every health problem, I'd seriously question the validity of that statement.

Storage at the Store. How are the supplements stored? Are they in a refrigerator when you buy them? Are they sitting on store shelves at room temperature? Although some probiotic strains do not need refrigeration, most do. Choose products that are stored in the refrigerator then store them in your fridge when you get them home. Try not to leave them in a hot vehicle for long. They might be fine for an hour or two but will have lost much of their potency if you leave them there for a weekend during the hot summer months.

Do Your Probiotics Contain What's on the Label?

Similar to other types of products, there is a big difference in quality among probiotic brands. ConsumerLab.com tested forty-one probiotic supplements manufactured by different companies. Here is an overview of their findings. The percentage indicates the number of CFUs a product actually contained compared to the amount claimed on the product:

Products that did *not* contain the number of CFUs specified on the label:

21st Century High Potency Acidophilus Probiotic Blend: Label indicates that the product contains "over 1 billion" probiotics, but testing showed it contained 179 million (17.9 percent).

Accuflora Advanced CD Probiotic: Label indicates that the product contains "over 1 billion," but testing showed it contained 191 to 383 million cells per two-caplet serving (19.2 percent).

Vitacost Probiotic: Label indicates that the product contains 35 billion probiotics, but testing showed it contained 5.7 billion, which is still significant but only 16.3 percent of the claimed amount.

Nature's Answer for Kids Probiotics: Label indicates that the product contains 5 billion cells per one-quarter teaspoon, but testing showed that it was 1.25 billion cells per one-quarter teaspoon of probiotic powder, or 24.9 percent of the claimed amount.

Nature's Plus Animal Parade AcidophiKidz: Berry Flavor indicates that it contains 1 billion cells "at the time of manufacture," but testing showed it contained 558 million cells per chewable capsule (55.8 percent).[27]

Of course, it is possible that these companies have improved their products or that there were issues with particular batches of the products used for testing.

Of the products tested by ConsumerLabs, here is a list of products that actually *contained the number of probiotics stated on the label*:

Align® Probiotic Supplement

Culturelle®

CVS/pharmacy® Probiotic Acidophilus

Dr. David Williams Probiotic Advantage

Dr. Mercola® Complete Probiotics

Enzymatic Therapy® Acidophilus Pearls™

Garden of Life® Raw Probiotics™ Ultimate Care

Jarrow Formulas® Jarro-Dophilus EPS®

Kyo-Dophilus®

Lee Swanson Genetic Designed Nutrition™ Ultimate Probiotic
   Formula

Metagenics® UltraFlora®

Nature Made®

Nature's Bounty® Advanced Probiotic

NOW® Gr8-Dophilus™

Nutri-Health® Flora Source Multi Probiotic® Capsules with
   Bif Relief 24–7™

Nutrition Now® PB 8®

Phillips® Colon Health® Probiotic Caps

Renew Life® Ultimate Flora™

Renew Life® Ultimate Flora Adult Formula

Renew Life® Ultimate Flora Critical Care

Rexall® Probiotic Acidophilus

Schiff® Digestive Advantage® Daily Probiotic

Sedona Labs® iFlora® Multi-Probiotics®

Solgar® Advanced Multi-Billion Dophilus®

Spring Valley® Probiotic Acidophilus

TruBiotics™

UAS Laboratories DDS® Plus 3

Do Your Probiotics Contain What's on the Label? (continued)

USANA® Probiotic

Vitacost® Probiotic 15–35

VSL#3®

Similar to Approved Product

Puritan's Pride® Probiotic 10: Similar to Nature's Bounty®
Advanced Priobiotic 10

Vitamin World® Probiotic: Similar to Nature's Bounty® Advanced
Priobiotic 10

Women's Product

RepHresh® Pro-B™

Senior's Product

Jarrow Formulas® Senior Jarro-Dophilus

Children's Products

Florastor® Kids

Nature's Answer® for Kids Probiotics

Nature's Plus® Animal Parade® AcidophiKidz®
Berry Flavor

Trunature® (Costco) Chewable Probiotic

Pet Products

Best Pet Health™ Probiotics with Wild Alaskan Salmon Oil for
Dogs and Cats

Only Natural Pet™ Probiotic Blend

Petco Digestive Enzymes and Probiotics for Dogs[28]

Obviously, there are many factors to consider when choosing a high-quality probiotic supplement. To help you cut through the clutter, on my website, I have listed some of the best probiotic supplements that I have personally used or recommended to my clients over the last twenty-five years. Additionally, I regularly share information about new advancements in probiotic research, testing, and production on my site to help you choose a product that is right for you. For more information about these probiotics, consult the Resources and Cutting-Edge Research sections at the back of this book and visit my website, www.TheProbioticPromise.com.

How to Take Probiotic Supplements for the Best Results

Probiotic supplements tend to work best over time. Do not expect to see immediate results like you would with certain other supplements, although I have witnessed almost immediate results when I have used probiotics to aid bloating, diarrhea, and indigestion. And my clients have reported the same almost-immediate results when using probiotics for these digestive issues.

Take probiotic supplements on an empty stomach (although adding them to smoothies and other foods is fine, as these types of foods tend to digest quickly and don't slow the probiotics from getting to the intestines where they ultimately need to be) and away from antibiotics or even natural products with antibiotic effects such as oregano oil, olive leaf, and similar supplements mentioned in Chapter 3. If you're taking antibiotics or herbal antibiotics, make sure you take your probiotics about two to three hours before or after. For most people the ideal time is either before bed or first thing in the morning. If you take it in the morning, try to leave at least twenty to thirty minutes before eating.

Most people benefit from two capsules or a half-teaspoon in the morning on an empty stomach. If you're taking probiotic powder, you can measure a half-teaspoon into water and drink it. Or add it to your smoothie.

Taking probiotic supplements on an empty stomach helps to ensure that they find their way past the digestive juices in the stomach, arriving intact in the small and large intestines. But you'll still benefit from adding probiotics to your smoothies, juices, or by eating them in yogurt or probiotic-rich cheeses (recipes at the back of this book), sauerkraut, or kimchi.

Whatever probiotic supplement you choose, it is important to drink plenty of water when taking them. That's because probiotics found in capsules or powders are basically inert until they are mixed with water. Make sure you're drinking plenty of water if you're eating probiotic-rich foods or taking probiotic supplements because, like you, the beneficial bacteria need water to function. The water rehydrates the bacteria, allowing them to become active so they can perform their many health-building functions. Once rehydrated, they work their magic in your intestines to help maintain or restore great health.

If you are suffering from a Candida infection, other type of infection, or a serious health condition, you may need a higher dose than if you're just taking probiotics for general health. Different conditions benefit from different probiotic strains, so there isn't really a "one-size-fits-all" probiotic that is ideal for all health problems, contrary to what some manufacturers might claim. I've offered the information in this book to help you sort through all the claims and find the right supplements for you. Unless you have a serious infection, start with the minimum dose recommended on the product label. If you have a serious infection, you should consult a health professional immediately and work with a naturally minded health practitioner who has extensive experience working with probiotics in this application.

Is It Safe and Recommended to Use Probiotics in the Vagina?

Some products are safe to use within the vagina to treat vaginal infections like bacterial or yeast overgrowth. In these cases choose a specific formula designed for this purpose. Either insert intravaginal suppositories, tablets, or capsules directly into the vagina or douche with a probiotic-water blend. For a douche, open the probiotic capsule and add to pure, unchlorinated water. Remember that chlorine kills beneficial bacteria, so chlorinated water should not be used for this purpose.

Which Probiotic Strains Are Best for You?

As you learned earlier, one strain of probiotic may be great to help you prevent or fight the flu but may not be as effective or therapeutic at all when trying to reduce high cholesterol levels. The following chart serves as a basic guideline to help you select the right probiotic for your specific health needs. It is based on the scientific evidence for using the particular strains to achieve therapeutic results. Keep in mind that the volume of research on probiotics grows almost daily, so there will always be new research that continues to expand our knowledge of the healing properties of various probiotics. The list on page 132 gives you a good start in choosing the probiotics that are best for you. Just match the probiotic to the condition.[29]

The Healing Power of Fermented Foods

As you'll discover in detail in the next chapter, different fermented foods contain different strains of probiotics. Because these cultures are typically airborne, there are also

Condition	Probiotic Strains Found in Research to Be Effective
Anxiety	*B. longum R0175* *L. bacillus helveticus R0052*
Cholesterol (high)	*L. reuteri NCIMB 30242* *E. faecium M-74*
Cold and flu	*L. plantarum HEAL9 (SDM 15312)* *L. paracasei 8700:2 (DSM 13434)* *L. acidophilus NCFM* *B. animalis lactis Bi-007*
Diarrhea resulting from antibiotic use, viral infection, or chemotherapy	*B. lactis Bi-07* *B. lactis BI-04* *L. GG* (in children) *L. reuteri* *L. casei* *L. bulgaricus* *S. thermophilus* *L. acidophilus* *L. acidophilus NCFM* *L. paracasei Lpc-37* *S. thermophilus* *S. boulardii*
H. pylori infection	Bifidobacterium Saccharomyces Lactobacillus
Irritable bowel syndrome	*B. infantis 35624* *B. lactis BB-12* *B. animalis* *L. GG* *L. reuteri DSM 17938* (children) *L. casei DG* *L. plantarum* *L. salivarius*
Periodontitis	*L. reuteri DSM 17938* *L. reuteri ATCC PTA 5289*
Traveler's diarrhea or food poisoning	*L. GG* *L. acidophilus* *L. bulgaricus* *S. thermophilus* *L. casei* *L. acidophilus NCFM* *L. paracasei Lpc-37* *B. lactis* *S. thermophilus* *S. boulardii*
Vaginal infections	*L. rhamnosus GR-1* *L. fermentum RC-14*

regional differences in the types of strains found in food products from foreign places. Some of the probiotic-rich foods include sauerkraut, miso, kimchi, and yogurt. Because there is a wide range of yogurt products on the market, ranging from great to completely unhealthy, let's take a closer look at these products.

Does Your Yogurt Contain Live Cultures?

Many commercially available brands of yogurt don't contain "live cultures." If you're choosing one, be sure to choose one that says "live cultures" on the label. Although the claim doesn't guarantee that the cultures are intact, it does increase the odds. If they are subjected to excessive heat during the manufacturing, processing, transportation, or storage of the products, the probiotic content will drop.

When yogurt contains live cultures it typically contains the bacteria *Lactobacillus acidophilus*, *Lactobacillus bulgaricus*, and sometimes strains of *Streptococcus salivarius* and Bifidobacteria. Because the cultures turn the milk sugar lactose into lactic acid, some people who are lactose intolerant can eat yogurt and not suffer the digestive distress they suffer from milk products. However, many people are actually allergic to dairy products. No amount of fermentation will enable these people to eat dairy-based yogurt without suffering. That's not to suggest that dairy yogurt is harmful. Like other allergies, dairy allergies are specific to individuals.

Although yogurt has many health benefits for some people, I don't consider dairy a health food. Researchers at Harvard University have questioned dairy as a part of our diet. It is possible to obtain all the benefits of yogurt from dairy-free yogurt with live cultures and avoid many of the inherent problems linked with dairy consumption.

Regardless of whether you choose dairy yogurt or dairy-free yogurt, the best way to ensure you're getting live cultures is to make it at home. Forget expensive machinery. Forget what you may have heard about making yogurt. It is easy, inexpensive, and can be done with no special equipment other than some probiotics.

Actually, learning how to make your own yogurt is a valuable skill not only because it tastes better than store-bought yogurt but also because you control all of the ingredients it contains. Further, it is more affordable than ready-made yogurt, and it is the only way to test your yogurt or probiotic powders and capsules to determine whether the cultures truly are alive. I included recipes for making various types of nondairy yogurt in the Recipe chapter at the back of this book. You can also make dairy yogurt the same way if you'd like.

How to Test Your Yogurt for Live Cultures

I wish I could tell you that there is a simple way to determine whether the yogurt you buy contains live cultures. The only true way of knowing whether your yogurt contains live cultures is to try making your own batch of yogurt from it. Although this process may take a bit of time while you wait for the cultures to work their magic, it is simple and easy. Here's how.

In a clean pot over low to medium heat, gently warm one quart (one liter) of milk of your choice (almond, coconut, soy, or cow's milk). If you're using almond milk, coconut, or soy milk, add a tablespoon of a sweetener such as honey; the yogurt won't have much of this sweetener left once it is cultured, as it is food for the probiotics. Once it is slightly warm but not hot—ideally, around 115 degrees—pour into a clean glass, ceramic bowl, or a crock. When the milk is lukewarm, add three tablespoons of yogurt and stir until combined. Place in a warm area where it will not be disturbed, and cover with a clean cloth. Allow to sit for eight to ten hours. The milk should have divided into a thick yogurt layer and a thin clearish-yellowish layer that forms the whey. Gently scoop out the thick yogurt into a bowl and reserve the whey so it can be used to make other fermented foods.

If the milk separated into the two layers mentioned, then your original yogurt contains live cultures. If it is still milk when you check it, there are no live cultures in the yogurt you're testing.

Five Yogurts That Have More Sugar Than Doughnuts Do

Most people assume that all yogurt is healthy. But that common misconception is causing people to ingest a lot more sugar than they bargained for. I reviewed many common brands of yogurt to determine how healthy they actually are. Here's a list of my five yogurt picks that have more sugar than doughnuts do (based on a Krispy Kreme doughnut, containing about ten grams of sugar each). I placed them in order based on the amount of sugar a six-ounce serving of yogurt contains, regardless of what serving size the package indicates, just to compare apples to apples. Of course, there are other nutritional factors to consider, so I'm not suggesting you eat doughnuts instead of yogurt.

Yoplait Strawberry Original Yogurt. A six-ounce package contains twenty-six grams of sugar. By comparison, a twelve-ounce can of Coke or Sprite (twice the amount) contains thirty-three grams of sugar. Ounce for ounce the Yoplait yogurt contains far more sugar than Coke.

Activia Blueberry Yogurt. Activia tied with Yoplait Strawberry Original for highest sugar content. Although it may appear at first glance to contain only nineteen grams of sugar (still high!), when you learn that amount is for a 4.4-ounce serving size, that means this yogurt contains

Five Yogurts That Have More Sugar Than Doughnuts Do (continued)

nearly twenty-six grams of sugar for a comparable 6-ounce serving size, or the equivalent of two and a half Krispy Kreme doughnuts.

Brown Cow Nonfat Vanilla. Contains twenty-five grams of sugar for a six-ounce serving size. That's also the equivalent of two and a half doughnuts.

Danone Fruit on the Bottom Yogurt, Blueberry. A six-ounce package of this yogurt contains twenty-four grams of sugar, or the equivalent of two and a half doughnuts.

Stonyfield Organic Smooth and Creamy French Vanilla. Contains 29 grams of sugar for a slightly larger eight-ounce serving, or the equivalent of 21.75 grams of sugar for a six-ounce serving, or just over two doughnuts.

So which yogurt should you choose? Choose either plain yogurt and add fresh fruit to it or choose Greek yogurt that tends to be naturally low in sugar. As an example, 100 grams of Danone Oikos Greek Yogurt contains 3.2 grams of sugar. Pay attention to both the grams of sugar number and the serving size, as some brands like Activia are actually much smaller than most others.

Marketing Gimmicks Disguised as Science

You may have noticed yogurt companies that claim to have exclusivity over specific strains of bacteria. As an example, let's look at "Bifidus Regularis" or "B. L. Regularis," which are trademarks owned by Compagnie Gervais Danone, or Dannon, or Danone, as it operates in the United States and Canada, respectively. The trademark can only be applied to words or phrases, not living creatures. Living creatures, including bacterial strains, cannot be patented either, as only processes are patented. Yet this trademark implies that the company's yogurt, namely, Activia, is the only source for an exclusive bacterial strain. On its website, television advertisements, and, presumably, elsewhere, Dannon states, "Activia is the only yogurt with the exclusive probiotic Bifidus Regularis®." But if you searched the company's trademark, you'd see that the US Patent and Trademark Office posted the disclaimer that "No claim is made to the exclusive right to use bifidus apart from the mark as shown." In other words, the company cannot make claims that they have a trademark on "bifidus" or the bacteria that bears the name.

If I didn't know this information, as a consumer I'd probably be more inclined to buy Activia over other products, believing that I'm getting an exclusive health-promoting bacterial strain. But I'm not. I'm simply getting a made-up name for a bacterial strain that is readily available in fermented foods and probiotic supplements. In my opinion, such a trademark and claim should not be allowable. I believe it is duping consumers. I'd never buy a product that dupes consumers, as I consider it an unethical business practice. I think consumers deserve to know the truth. Such trademarks and claims are simply slick marketing, not nutritional science. If you see any product that claims to contain an exclusive strain of bacteria, it is important to know that the claim is not true. It is merely marketing mumbo-jumbo.

Additionally, the made-up name this company uses, "Bifidus Regularis®" or "B. L. Regularis," sounds like either a *Bifidobacterium* or *Lactobacilli* (*B.* or *L.*), and it just causes confusion in the marketplace. The actual name for Bifidus Regularis is *Bifidobacterium animalis DN-173 010*.[30]

According to ConsumerLabs.com, "Advertising claims on Activia (as well as related DanActive drinks) indicating them to be 'clinically proven' and 'scientifically proven' to aid digestion have been (or are being) modified to read 'clinical studies show' as a result of lawsuits in the U.S. and Canada."

Marketing Gimmicks Disguised as Science (continued)

If you want to ensure that your yogurt includes *Bifidus lactis*, which is the reported strain in Activia, make your own yogurt using a high-quality probiotic supplement or powder that contains this strain, which will help to colonize your yogurt and impart any associated beneficial health effects. Also, it is the only way to ensure that any yogurt or probiotic cultures are truly alive. I discuss step-by-step instructions on how to make your own dairy-free yogurt in the following chapter. Once you've tried homemade you'll probably always want it on hand.

Chapter 6

Fall in Love with Fermented Foods

"Industrially produced food is dead. It severs our connection to the life forces that sustain us and deprives us of our access to the powerful magic so abundantly present in the natural world."

—Sandor Ellix Katz, *Wild Fermentation*

Jordan Improves His Sun-Damaged Skin

Jordan, a forty-nine-year-old man, came to see me to address scarring from sun damage. Because skin cancer ran in his family and he had so much sun damage from unprotected skin and severe sunburns as a child, he was worried about getting skin cancer. He had severe scarring on his skin, and some areas showed signs of raised growths.

I encouraged him to get tested for skin cancer and, in the meantime, suggested we explore dietary improvements and a few supplements to give his body a much-needed boost to help his skin heal.

After reviewing Jordan's diet diary, I learned that it was surprisingly healthy. It was primarily plant-based with some chicken, high in

Jordan Improves His Sun-Damaged Skin

vegetables, low in sugar, low in dairy products, and even included legumes on a daily basis. He ate organic foods as much as possible and, with the exception of the sun damage from his childhood years, he seemed to be in great health.

I asked him to start eating fermented foods, preferably at every meal. He began making his morning smoothies with vegan yogurt (I gave him my recipe that you'll find at the back of the book), drank kombucha before his lunch or dinner meal, and added sauerkraut or another type of pickled vegetable to at least one meal daily. He even faithfully made and ate my probiotic-rich nondairy cheeses (for which you'll find similar recipes at the back of this book).

We also added more anticancer foods like those I gave Wes (see page 16) to his diet and added a few supplements, including vitamin A drops, curcumin (an extract from the spice turmeric), resveratrol (an extract from grapes), and alpha lipoic acid (an excellent antioxidant). I also gave him an ointment made from the anticancer herb pokeroot and coconut oil. I knew it would take some time to notice the change in sun damage because he'd had it for many years, so I suggested he come back to see me in three months and, if he needed more guidance, to come in earlier than that.

Because his diet and lifestyle were already so healthy, Jordan found it easy to stick to the program. And clearly he did. When he came back in a few months to see me his skin already looked significantly improved—I'd estimate about 50 percent reduced in discoloration. He said the damaged areas were also less itchy. He also pointed out the spots where a couple of growths had been but had fallen off. That's not to say that fermented foods are the antidote to sun damage but that when we give our bodies the healing foods they need, they are more capable of healing us. Jordan also mentioned that he hadn't realized how much bloating he had in the past, but since he began eating more fermented foods he noticed he didn't feel bloated anymore. This is something I regularly hear from clients to whom I've recommended more fermented foods.

As a child, I often visited my grandparents at their large farm an hour from my home in southern Ontario. They had a massive field of corn devoted to food for their animals. Additionally, they had a two-acre fruit and vegetable garden to feed their nine children, one of whom was my dad. Whenever I visited them my grandmother asked me to go out to the garden to pick beans, raspberries, strawberries, kohlrabi, and many other fruits and vegetables. I was always an independent sort of person and was thrilled to spend hours at a time on my own in their lush garden, picking whatever was in season. The raspberry bushes alone were taller than I was until I was a teenager. At the height of the season the corn stood at least ten feet tall. As a child, it felt like being in a jungle in an exotic place, and I loved it.

I especially loved raspberry picking, or should I say, raspberry eating? They were the same thing to me. I ate a raspberry for every one that made its way into my basket. After picking the produce I brought it back to my grandparents' kitchen, where my grandmother made almost everything from scratch from fresh, mostly farm-grown foods straight from their garden. As soon as the produce was picked it was either made into a meal or preserved and stored in their massive root cellar.

My grandmother made a wide range of fermented foods as well, including cucumber pickles, bean pickles, sauerkraut, and dandelion wine. The kitchen was always a hub of activity as she prepared the food for her nine children and, later, their spouses, and sixteen grandchildren when they visited. My grandfather's influence was also apparent. Born in Austria, he came to North America when he was a small boy with his mother, sister, and a tradition of fermented foods that he later taught to my grandmother, who kept the sauerkraut and fermented food tradition alive in my family.

My grandparents knew that their food growing and preservation techniques were also keeping their family healthy, although the term *probiotics* wasn't in their (or anyone else's) vocabulary at that time. They knew that they were preserving food at the height of their nutritional goodness and that their food-preservation techniques seemed to add to the healthfulness of the foods. They realized that these fermented foods and fermentation techniques were passed down from generation to generation for a reason— they improved peoples' health. My grandparents were among the many parents, grandparents, and other ancestors who used fermentation as a part of their daily lives.

This tradition began thousands of years ago. Somehow these ancient people instinctively fermented foods as a method of preservation and as a way to improve their health. The earliest records of fermentation date back to 5400 BC with wine making in Iran. Babylonians started the fermentation of milk in 5000 BC to create yogurt; the Chinese began fermenting cabbage in 4000 BC; Egyptians used "leaven," which is now known as yeast, to raise bread dough as early as 3000 BC; and native peoples of North America made one of the earliest alcoholic beverages in the area we now call Mexico around 2000 BC. Most of these people hadn't even heard of bacteria yet, as bacteria were a more recent discovery, but somehow they figured out how to ferment foods and that the culturing process improved the health benefits of the foods they ate. In 76 AD Roman historian Plinio indicated that fermented milk helped GI infections. Early voyagers like Roman emperor Tiberius in the first century AD to Captain James Cook (no relation) in the eighteenth century, who sailed the seas in search of

Food Traditions and Their Origins

Germans and other Central Europeans have sauerkraut; Japanese have miso, rice wine, soy sauce and tamari, and vegetable pickles; Koreans have kimchi and other pickled vegetables; Greeks have olives and yogurt; Italians have olives, cured meats, and wine; Indians have chutney; Australians have Vegemite; Scandinavians have pickled fish; and most cultures, including North Americans, have some variations on sourdough bread and pickles. Of course, there are many others, but these are some of the main fermented food traditions still employed worldwide.

new lands, took fermented cabbage to protect their crews from intestinal infections and diseases, including scurvy, which is the result of a vitamin C deficiency.[1] Other sailors who hadn't determined the health benefits of sauerkraut often suffered serious disease or even death.

In modern times around the world people make many types of fermented foods such as yogurt, sauerkraut, cheeses, miso, kombucha, ginger beer, beer, wine, kimchi, vinegar, and many other foods and beverages. Fortunately, many of these traditions are still alive and play a large role in the various cultures where they originate.

The previous chapter showed you how to select the best probiotics for your health and wellness; the next two chapters show you how to get probiotics into your diet from the food you eat.

Types of Fermentation

There are many different types of fermentation processes, which can differ significantly from each other, but here is some of what the main ones involve.

Brining

Brine is simply a saltwater solution that is poured over vegetables (sometimes meat or fish). The salt not only makes the food tender but also it prevents harmful bacteria from accessing the food, thereby giving the probiotic organisms an opportunity to take over and transform the food. It is the primary technique involved in creating sauerkraut, naturally fermented pickles, and other fermented vegetables. The process usually involves leaving the food undisturbed for a week or more until it becomes a probiotic-rich food. You'll find recipes involving the brining technique in the Recipe section.

Addition of Probiotic Powders

You can easily ferment foods like dairy milk or nut or seed milk into yogurt or cheeses using probiotic powders or the probiotic powder within capsules found in the refrigerator section of most health food stores. The process differs slightly depending on the food but usually involves emptying the contents of two or three probiotic capsules or adding a teaspoon of the powder to whatever food you're trying to ferment, then leaving it in a warm place for eight hours or more. You'll find recipes involving probiotic powders in the Recipe section.

Yogurt Starter

Some foods can be fermented simply with the addition of a few tablespoons of either store-bought or homemade yogurt with live cultures. This is an easy way to make a new batch of yogurt. Although it has traditionally been used to make dairy yogurt, I use this method every few days to make a new batch of nondairy yogurt from almond, cashew, soy, or coconut milk. You'll find a yogurt recipe using leftover yogurt from another batch in the Recipe section.

Whey as Starter

In the same way that a few tablespoons of yogurt can be saved to make a new batch of yogurt, the clear liquid byproduct of yogurt making, called "whey," can be saved to make new batches of yogurt. Additionally, it can be saved as a starter culture for making other types of foods, including many different fermented vegetable dishes. You can also add the whey to smoothies, salad dressings, soups, and sauces to make them healthier and full of probiotics. You'll find a yogurt recipe using leftover whey from yogurt making in the Recipe section. You can also add a half cup of whey to almost any brine recipe as a way to give the probiotics a head start at culturing the food.

Alcoholic Fermentation

Yeasts ferment grains, potatoes, grapes, or sugarcane, among other foods, in an environment absent of oxygen to make beer, wine, and other alcoholic beverages. In this process the yeasts produce alcohol (ethanol) and carbon dioxide. Although some of these beverages contain beneficial probiotics, the alcohol, carbon dioxide, and yeasts may present challenges to the body when drunk frequently.

Vinegar Fermentation

Similar to alcoholic ferments, vinegar is formed when the alcohol is exposed to oxygen and in the presence of a group of bacteria called Acetobacter, which convert alcohol into acetic acid, or vinegar. You may have experienced this process if you've ever left a bottle of wine open for a long period of time. Some examples of this acetic acid–type of fermentation include apple cider vinegar, red or white wine vinegar, and coconut vinegar. If kombucha tea is fermented for longer than the desired length of time, it can turn into vinegar because the kombucha culture contains the Acetobacter bacteria; however, if you want a green tea vinegar, this lengthier culturing time may be desirable.

Sodium-Rich Fermentation Pastes

This process usually involves grains or legumes that are cooked and mashed to form a paste, along with added salt, to create soy sauce, miso, and other primarily Asian fermented foods. This process can take many months, so I have not included recipes to make miso or soy sauce; however, there are many excellent probiotic-rich products on the market, and I encourage you to try different ones. I have included a delicious recipe for a Ginger Vinaigrette on page 206 in the Recipe section of this book to help you explore new ways to use miso.

Although there are other types of fermentation processes, these are the most commonly used and familiar ones. We'll discuss many of the health benefits of these different types of fermented foods throughout this chapter, along with the exciting research that shows how these foods can transform our health. If you thought fermented foods were a thing of the past or just

Sourdough: A Probiotic Food or Not?

The history of sourdough breads goes back approximately six thousand years.[2] Sourdough breads rise as a result of "sour dough" that has captured naturally occurring yeasts in the air to transform ground grains and water into a starter culture. Not only does it leaven the bread with which it is made, but it also adds that uniquely sourdough-like taste. Keep in mind that most sourdough breads now are made via commercial processes that don't actually involve "sour dough" at all. A sourdough starter can be saved to make a new batch of bread. Because the air can contain different types of yeasts, sourdough breads tend to taste different from one place to another. That's how San Francisco sourdough bread has its own unique flavor not found elsewhere. Although sourdough breads tend to be preferable to those made with commercial yeast and are usually more digestible and nutritious, keep in mind that sourdough breads are not probiotic-rich foods because the beneficial microorganisms are killed during the baking process.

helpful for gut health, you'll want to explore more of them. They are delicious and nutritious but really warrant consideration for their widespread healing abilities that go well beyond the gut.

The Straight Goods on Yogurt

Yogurt is perhaps the most widely known and widely used fermented food in North America. The word *yogurt* is derived from the Turkish word *yogurt*, but because it is eaten in nations around the world and has been for so many years, the exact origin of yogurt is unknown.

Yogurt appears in ancient Indian and Persian records, but the oldest writings are attributed to Pliny the Elder, who wrote that some "barbarous nations" could "thicken the milk into a substance with an agreeable acidity." Yogurt has also been a part of the Russian, Western Asian, and Southeastern and Central European cultures for many years. Russian Nobel laureate and biologist Ilya Ilyich Mechnikov believed that regular consumption of yogurt was responsible for the unusually long life spans of Bulgarian peasants. Mechnikov may have been correct. More and more research on yogurt's health benefits indicates it may be helpful for many conditions and in preventing additional health concerns.

Metabolic Syndrome. Scientists have found that yogurt cultured with *L. plantarum* improved cholesterol levels, blood sugar levels, and homocysteine levels in women with metabolic syndrome.[3] Metabolic syndrome is a cluster of four conditions, including increased blood pressure, a high blood sugar level, excess body fat around the waist, and abnormal cholesterol levels. When these symptoms occur together doctors diagnose metabolic syndrome, which increases a person's risk of heart disease, stroke, and diabetes.[4] Excessively high levels of homocysteine can result in damage to the arteries, the brain, and the body's genetic material (DNA) and can increase the risk for over fifty diseases, including Alzheimer's disease, cancer, depression, diabetes, heart attack, stroke, and rheumatoid arthritis.[5] Reducing homocysteine levels, such as through yogurt consumption, is an important factor in preventing these serious conditions.

Respiratory Infections. Research has also explored the effects of yogurt cultured with the probiotic *L. casei DN-114001* on the duration of respiratory infections in the elderly. The results were impressive: the fermented yogurt significantly reduced the average duration of respiratory infection. The elderly participants taking the fermented yogurt with live cultures also had fewer respiratory infections and less nasal congestion than the placebo group.[6]

Phytonutrient Absorption. Yogurt consumption also increases nutrient absorption even from other foods eaten at the same meal. A recent study found that yogurt consumption increased the absorbability of the phytonutrients called isoflavones found in soy milk when the two foods were eaten at the same morning meal. This is good news for postmenopausal women, many of whom experience lower levels of the hormone estrogen and, as a result, are at an increased risk for a variety of health conditions, including heart disease and osteoporosis.[7] Isoflavones are Nature's hormone replacement therapy, which can reduce many of the health issues women experience during and after menopause. I will discuss iso-flavones and their many additional health benefits momentarily.

Cancer. Eating yogurt with certain live cultures has also been shown to have anticancer effects. In particular, the specific probiotic strain *Lactobacillus casei CRL 431* tested on mice with breast tumors showed blocked tumor development or delayed tumor growth, improved immune response so the body could attack the tumor, and a decreased number of blood vessels feeding the tumor, all of which were beneficial in fighting the breast cancer.[8] Although further research is needed to explore the anticancer effects of yogurt consumption on humans, this study suggests yogurt with this particular *L. casei* strain has potential anticancer benefits.

H. pylori **infection.** Yogurt is also demonstrating great potential in the treatment of the *H. pylori* infection (discussed in detail in Chapter 3, pages 64–66), which has been linked to ulcers, gastritis, and cancer of the glandular or lymphatic tissues in the body.[9] Studies have explored the effects of yogurt with live cultures on *H. pylori* infections as a possible complementary therapy for treating this infection. They found a significant beneficial effect of yogurt consumption in eradicating *H. pylori*, suggesting value in the regular consumption of yogurt and even doctors' prescriptive use of yogurt in treating *H. pylori* infections and related health conditions.[10]

Food Poisoning. Certain strains of probiotics used during the fermentation process may actually help prevent spoilage and reduce the likelihood of experiencing food poisoning. Yogurt fermented with the probiotic strain *Lactobacillus paracasei CBA L74* was found to protect against Salmonella infections and may protect against the formation of colitis. Scientists have found that *L. paracasei*–fermented yogurt inhibited the body's release of cytokines, inflammatory compounds, while increasing anti-inflammatory compounds. They concluded that these results may offer benefits for infant nutrition because the fermented milk could be used in infant formula, providing immune system benefits for the infants without carrying harmful bacteria like Salmonella, which could be dangerous to an immature infant immune system.[11]

Brain Health. According to research presented in the journal *Nutritional Neuroscience*, consuming whey, which is the clearish liquid byproduct of yogurt production, can improve learning and memory in mice.[12] The whey used in the study contained the probiotic *L. helveticus*. This cutting-edge research suggests a possible link between brain health, learning and memory, and probiotics.

"But I Eat Yogurt"

Over the years I've heard many health aficionados tell me that they get all the probiotics they need from eating yogurt daily.

Although it is true that a good-quality yogurt contains some naturally occurring probiotics that confer health benefits, many do not. Even yogurt that contains live cultures typically has only a couple of strains of bacteria. And, as you learned in the previous chapters, there are health reasons to obtain many more than that. For example, the flu protection conferred by eating kimchi is the result of consuming *Lactobacillus plantarum DK119* naturally present in the Korean condiment. Although yogurt may have some beneficial strains of probiotics, it simply doesn't contain this antiviral strain. That's just one example.

Another reason that eating yogurt may not be sufficient is that the cultures tend to become depleted over time, particularly if the temperatures increase during transportation or storage. Although yogurt may have started with live cultures, they rarely contain the same numbers by the time they get to consumers.

Alternatives to Dairy Yogurt

Fortunately, there are many delicious natural alternatives to cow's milk yogurt, including coconut, soy, and almond yogurt. If you purchase them in a store, be sure to check for "live cultures" either on the ingredient list or somewhere on the package. You can purchase these at health food stores and, increasingly, more mainstream grocery stores. You can also make your own. (For more on this, see page 186.)

We discussed the research on the health benefits of dairy yogurt, but there is also a growing body of research showing that the regular consumption of soy yogurt, also called fermented soy milk, confers a wide range of health benefits, including improving heart health, reducing cholesterol and triglycerides, balancing hormones, improving nutrition, reducing inflammation, and even offering anticancer benefits.

The Problems with Most Dairy Products

When yogurt contains live cultures it may actually improve the digest-ibility of the milk from which it was made. That means that some people who are lactose intolerant can eat dairy-based yogurt without the typical digestive complaints dairy products cause. However, be aware that dairy products may not be suitable as part of a healthy diet and are certainly not right for all people, for a variety of reasons, including:[13]

1. Dairy products are mucous forming and can contribute to ear infections. I've had countless clients that I've advised to stop eating dairy products as a way to heal their ear infections. And it has worked time after time.

2. Cow's milk is intended for baby cows. We're the only spe-cies (other than those we domesticate) that drinks milk after infancy. And we're definitely the only species drinking the milk of a different species. Baby cows have four stomachs to digest milk. We have one.

3. Dairy products contain hormones. Not only are the naturally present hormones in cow's milk stronger than human hor-mones, but the animals are also routinely given steroids and other hormones to plump them up and increase their milk production. These hormones can negatively affect our delicate human hormonal balance.

4. Most cows are fed inappropriate food. Commercial feed for cows contains all sorts of ingredients, including genetically modified corn, genetically modified soy, animal products, chicken manure, cottonseed, pesticides, and antibiotics. Guess what that feed becomes? The milk you drink.

5. Pesticides in cow feed find their way into the milk and dairy products that we consume. Pesticides are neurotoxins that can be harmful to our bodies.

6. Most dairy products are pasteurized to kill potentially harmful bacteria. During the pasteurization process, vitamins, proteins, and enzymes are also destroyed. Enzymes assist with the digestion process, and when these enzymes are destroyed the milk becomes harder to digest, therefore putting a strain on our bodies' enzyme systems.

7. Most milk is homogenized, which denatures the milk's proteins, making it harder to digest. Many peoples' bodies react to these proteins as though they are "foreign invaders," causing their immune systems to overreact.

8. Research shows that the countries whose citizens consume the most dairy products have the highest incidence of osteoporosis, contrary to what dairy bureaus try to tell us.

9. Research links dairy products with the formation of arthritis.

Although there are many issues with milk consumption due to the commercialization and degradation of milk during production, there is a large body of evidence to support the consumption of yogurt made with high-quality, preferably organic milk. I, personally, prefer non-dairy yogurt and find that it is superior for my health, but obviously the choice is yours to make.

Heart Health. According to a study assessing soy yogurt's ability to reduce some of the key indicators for heart disease such as blood cholesterol and triglyceride levels as well as liver cholesterol and triglyceride levels, this fermented food is proving itself to be a heart health superfood. Researchers in Japan found that animals eating soy milk fermented with *Bifidobacterium* probiotics—soy yogurt—had reduced levels of all of the above markers of heart disease and even reduced total blood cholesterol levels by 20 percent in six weeks.[14] The exact amount needed to obtain these results in humans is still to be determined, but daily consumption of soy yogurt is likely to assist with reducing cholesterol and triglycerides and overall heart health.

And it appears it is never too late to start benefiting from soy yogurt's heart-healing effects. A Russian study observed the effects of consuming soy yogurt for thirty days on men and women aged thirty-eight to sixty-nine years who had already had heart attacks. Those that ate the soy yogurt had a 36.3 percent decrease in cholesterol levels, compared to only 24.7 percent decrease in people not eating the yogurt. The researchers concluded that the soy yogurt had a significant strengthening effect on the effectiveness of basic therapy after heart attacks and suggested that those who had suffered from a heart attack should include soy yogurt early in their rehabilitation programs.[15] Anything that shows such promise for heart disease prevention and treatment is a welcome natural option, especially because heart disease is the number one killer in the United States and Canada. Other research in the *Journal of Science and Food Agriculture* showed that regular consumption of soy yogurt fermented with *L. plantarum* or *Streptococcus thermophilus* relaxed the vascular system.[16]

Cancer. Soy yogurt with live cultures is showing potential in the treatment of colon cancer as well. Researchers studied the anticancer effects of fermenting soy milk with the probiotics *S. thermophilus* and *B. infantis* into yogurt. They found that the fermentation process decreased cancer cells' ability to proliferate and increased the antitumor effect of the soy.[17]

Soy yogurt may also have anticancer benefits that go beyond the digestive tract. Scientists in Malaysia have found that soy yogurt fermented with several probiotic cultures, including *L. acidophilus*, *L. casei*, *Bifidobacterium*, and *B. longum* as well as prebiotics like FOS, inulin, and others, had beneficial effects that, according to the study authors, could "reduce the risks of hypertension and hormone-dependent diseases such as breast cancer, prostate cancer, and osteoporosis."[18]

Osteoporosis. This condition is characterized by low bone mass or loss of bone mass over time. The bones lose their minerals, become porous, and are vulnerable to fractures or breaks. According to some estimates, in the United States alone 10 million people, mostly women, suffer from osteoporosis. Although we tend to think of it as a disease of insufficient calcium intake, there is research that indicates that those nations with the highest calcium intake also have the highest incidence of osteoporosis.[19] Although calcium definitely plays a role, there are many other possible factors at work, one of which may be probiotic consumption and gut health. The Malaysian study is not the only one that shows soy yogurt consumption may help stave off osteoporosis; multiple other studies demonstrate the anti-osteoporotic effects in animals of consuming soy yogurt rich in probiotics.

The Next Antiaging Cosmetic? In a study at the Department of Food and Nutrition at the College of Human Ecology, Yonsei University, in Seoul, South Korea, researchers assessed the effects of fermented soy milk's therapeutic effects on low-grade inflammatory diseases, particularly in the skin of the animals tested. They found that soy yogurt could prevent skin inflammation when it replaced dairy products in the animals' diets. It appeared to have this effect by reducing the expression of the genes involved in creating skin inflammation.[20] But eating the fermented soy milk was not the only way the probiotic cultures improved skin health in animals. In another study researchers found that applying soy yogurt cultured with Bifidobacteria for six weeks to the animals' skin resulted in significant improvement in elasticity and hydration. The scientists expect that the fermented soy will become a new cosmetic ingredient to prevent the loss of skin elasticity associated with wrinkling.[21]

Soy and Prebiotics. Compounds naturally found in soy milk and soybeans have been found to act as food for beneficial bacteria—*prebiotics*. Researchers found that various natural sugars found in soy called oligosaccharides, raffinose, and stachyose were food for Bifidobacteria (except *Bifidobacteria bifidum*, which for some unknown reason did not use these compounds as food) but could not be used by disease-causing bacteria like *E. coli* and *Clostridium* bacteria.[22] So if you were wondering how it is possible to make soy yogurt with beneficial bacteria while keeping harmful bacteria at bay during the culturing process, their research answers the question. First, the addition of beneficial bacteria by emptying the probiotic capsules inoculates the soy milk with good bacteria, giving them a head start. Then, the natural sugars found in the soy milk (along with some extras I suggest you use in the recipes in Chapter 7) encourage the growth of the good bacteria but are not used by the harmful ones, further allowing the good bacteria to crowd out or, perhaps more accurately, starve out harmful bacteria that may be present in any food. This is the premise by which harmful bacteria are crowded out of other foods during the fermentation process as well.

If you're worried about eating these sugars in your diet, you need not. They act as the food for the beneficial bacteria and leave little left in the food, so provided the soy yogurt or other food is adequately fermented, there won't be much, if any, natural sugars present in the food you eat. But there will be high amounts of probiotics that proliferate thanks to the naturally present sugars.

Making your own dairy-free yogurt is easier than you might think. I make it every week and usually multiple times a week. You'll find my recipes for Dairy-Free Yogurt and Sweet Yogurt in the Recipe section at the back of this book. It is just as delicious as dairy yogurt, although you may find the taste is different depending on the type of "milk" you use. I've successfully made yogurt from all of these types of dairy-free "milks"; however, I wouldn't say that they were all equal in results. Soy milk tends to work well for yogurt. Almond milk tends to be a bit thin and results in a delicious-tasting yogurt, albeit a fairly small amount considering the amount of milk used. Experiment with different types until you find the one or ones you like the best. If almond yogurt isn't for you, try soy yogurt (made with only certified organic soy milk, as soy tends to be heavily genetically modified). I also included a recipe for yogurt made with almonds and cashews to help you reap the benefits of these nuts along with the probiotic benefits of yogurt. It is high in calcium, magnesium, and healthy fats.

The Great Soy Debate

The culturing process of turning soy milk into soy yogurt appears to increase its nutritional benefits. The same researchers at Yonsei University, in Seoul, South Korea, found that the fermented soy had more cancer-fighting, heart health–boosting, and hormone-balancing isoflavones than did the unfermented soy. Although soy milk and cultured soy milk, or soy yogurt, naturally contain the phytonutrients known as isoflavones, which can be valuable to women as Nature's own estrogen replacement therapy, the fermentation process appears to increase the bioavailability of these beneficial substances. Isoflavones are natural plant hormones that play an important role in regulating human hormones, particularly during perimenopause, the ten years prior to menopause, menopause, and the postmenopausal years. Isoflavones have been also shown in research to reduce the incidence of hormone-related cancers like breast and prostate cancer.

There is a lot of misinformation regarding isoflavones and soy out there, particularly on the Internet, due to their ability to function like weak estrogens in our bodies. Even many health practitioners are misguided about isoflavones. Let me try to set the record straight.

Genistein is one of the key isoflavones found in soy products and is the most like human estrogen of all the isoflavones found in soy. It can actually help to balance our bodies' estrogen levels, whether we have too much or too little estrogen. That's because when our bodies have too much estrogen and we ingest weak plant estrogens in the form of genistein, these can bind to the receptors and stop our bodies from producing more estrogen, or prevent our body's own estrogen, which is much stronger, from binding to these sites. Because plant estrogens are weaker, they can help lower our estrogen levels. Conversely, if we do not have enough estrogen, ingesting more through foods like soy yogurt helps to increase the amount of estrogen in our bodies.

Genistein's hormonal-balancing role couldn't be more important. We are currently exposed to synthetically produced xenoestrogens, primarily from plastics and other environmental toxins. Once inside our bodies these synthetic estrogens, which are much stronger than our bodies' own estrogen, can wreak havoc. Some experts estimate that many xenoestrogens may be one hundred times stronger than our own hormones. These synthetic hormone mimickers disrupt our delicate hormonal systems. (For more information on xenoestrogens, consult my book *Weekend Wonder Detox*.) When we eat soy foods and the genistein they contain, it binds to hormone receptor sites, preventing synthetic xenoestrogens from plastics and other chemicals from floating around our bloodstream where they can do damage.

Genistein has many other health benefits, including preventing free radical damage in our bodies. It also has anticancer properties and has been shown to be helpful with metabolic syndrome, a prediabetic condition and an underlying factor in obesity for many people. It has also been proven helpful in preventing heart attacks and strokes by acting as an anticlotting agent.[23]

Many doctors tell people to avoid genistein if they are at risk for hormone-related cancers (particularly breast and prostate cancer), but research shows that consuming isoflavones like genistein may actually protect against these forms of cancer.[24] Many doctors assume that because synthetic estrogen taken in drug form can aggravate hormone-related cancers, the same must be true of plant estrogens like genistein. But plants are far more "intelligent" than the synthetic compounds we manufacture in a laboratory setting. Plants naturally contain hundreds or even thousands of compounds, many of which work synergistically to aid our healing, whereas drugs are single ingredients synthesized in a laboratory. And as you learned earlier, the weak plant hormones can bind to hormone receptor sites and prevent the body's production of excess and more potent estrogens, thereby helping to restore balance regardless of whether these hormones are high or low.

Some people express concern about compounds in soy that block the absorption of certain nutrients like iron. Research has found that the fermentation process of turning soy milk into soy yogurt significantly reduced the content of the antinutrient compounds, rendering them insignificant.[25] Other research found that the fermentation of soy milk into soy yogurt using *L. acidophilus*, *L. bulgaricus*, *L. casei*, *L. plantarum*, and *L. fermentum* along with the yeast *S. boulardii* improved the bioavailability of isoflavones, assisted in the digestion of protein, provided more calcium, enhanced intestinal health, and supported the immune system all while decreasing the antinutrient phytic acid and increasing the availability of minerals.

Men and Soy

I've heard many men express concern about eating soy products due to the possible hormonal effects and their resulting worry about the hormones' effect on sexual health and potency. Remember our hormone receptor discussion above? It applies to men as well. And it is particularly true when it comes to fermented soy. Men might find an animal study published in the journal *Applied Physiology, Nutrition, and Metabolism* interesting. Scientists assessed the effects of rats' consumption of fermented soy yogurt. Because wheel running is thought to reflect the equivalent of voluntary exercise in humans, the amount of wheel running was measured in animals eating the soy yogurt compared to those that did not. The animals that ate the soy yogurt voluntarily engaged in significantly more wheel running and sexual activity than the rats that didn't eat the soy yogurt.[26] Although no study has been done on men who consume soy yogurt to see how much more voluntary exercise and sexual activity they may participate in, it is likely that the study results translate to human males as well.

What You Need to Know About Kefir

Most people know about the health benefits of yogurt, but few have even heard about kefir (pronounced ke-FEER). In many ways it is like a drinkable form of yogurt, but it offers even greater health benefits than yogurt. Like yogurt, kefir is typically a cultured milk product, although there are nondairy and juice varieties as well, that has a tart, tangy, somewhat sour taste and a slightly bubbly characteristic.

Kefir comes from the Turkish word "keif," which means "good feeling," probably for the health benefits it offers. This beverage originates in the Caucasus Mountains in Eastern Europe.[27] Slightly thinner in consistency than yogurt, it is made with kefir grains, which aren't actually grains but a combination of various bacteria and yeasts. Some commercial kefir products are made with powdered kefir starter, which isn't truly authentic. Like yogurt, many commercial, bottled kefir products are frequently heavily sweetened and flavored, so be sure to read the labels if you're buying premade kefir.

It's believed that, on average, kefir typically contains three times the overall number of probiotics than yogurt and about ten to twenty different bacteria and yeast strains.[28]

Vitamin Boost. Kefir naturally contains several B-complex vitamins, including thiamine, folic acid, riboflavin, and biotin.[29] Additionally, the live cultures manufacture vitamin B_{12}, which is also known as the "energy vitamin" because it boosts cellular and overall energy. Kefir also naturally contains magnesium, calcium, phosphorus, and vitamin K.

Digestion and Immunity Boost. In studies, kefir has been shown to improve digestibility of milk, even for many lactose-intolerant individuals. Other research shows that kefir can prevent or treat some digestive concerns and boost immunity to illness. Many people report that drinking kefir on a daily basis shows digestive improvements within a week or two.

Other Conditions. Research shows that Kefir consumption reduced cholesterol levels, lowered blood glucose levels, and prevented blood pressure spikes in animals.[30] Other studies suggest that kefir and its constituents have antimicrobial, antitumor, anticarcinogenic, and immune system–regulating activity.[31] As if that weren't enough, kefir consumption may offer hope for allergy, asthma, and colitis sufferers as well as overweight, obese, and diabetic individuals.[32] Still further research showed that regular kefir consumption enhanced the immune system's ability to fight off viruses and parasites, such as Giardia—a common cause of abdominal cramps, bloating, nausea, and diarrhea that usually results from drinking contaminated water while traveling.[33] Kefir has also shown potential for preventing or treating fatty liver disease, which is a common factor in weight that won't budge as well as diabetes.[34]

Cancer. New research has showed that probiotics found in some kefir products hold promise in treating cancer. One type of probiotic called *Lactobacillus kefiri P-IF* was shown to help destroy human leukemia cells, even when multiple cancer drugs were unable to induce the cancer cell–killing process. The scientists concluded that the novel kefir bacteria "may act as a potential therapy for the treatment of multidrug-resistant leukemia."[35]

Diabetes. Kefir consumption also presents new possibilities in managing diabetes. Research in the journal *Nitric Oxide* found that kefir administered to diabetic animals for eight weeks resulted in significant improvement in many of the measurements linked to diabetes, including blood sugar, C-reactive protein, and measure of kidney health. Diabetes is frequently associated with abnormalities in kidney function, so the results suggest excellent prospects for the use of kefir in treating diabetes and to delay the progression of diabetic complications.[36]

If you are purchasing kefir products, beware of added flavors and sugars. Kefir is easy to make on an ongoing basis, so you can keep a regular supply to boost your health. And homemade kefir is far superior to most of the bottled varieties. It takes a couple of minutes to add the "grains"—the bacteria and yeasts—to the milk, dairy-free milk, or juice you're using and then twenty-four to forty-eight hours to ferment. Because probiotic cultures tend to dwindle over time during storage, making your own is also a good way to ensure the integrity of the probiotic cultures in your kefir. I recommend using kefir grains over starter powder for a more authentic kefir that is full of live cultures. You can drink kefir on its own, stir in vanilla or cocoa for a flavored beverage, add it to your breakfast cereal, or add fruit and whip it into a delicious smoothie.

Magic Miso

Miso is a fermented food, typically made from soybeans, although I've seen rice and chickpea miso as well. Most people are only aware of miso's use in making miso soup; however, there are other ways miso is used as a flavoring, such as in salad dressings. It is a staple food in the Japanese diet, but a similar type of fermented soy is used in other cultures as well.

Miso is rich in vitamins, minerals, plant proteins, carbohydrates (the "good carbs"), enzymes, and, of course, probiotics. It has even been referred to as a medicinal food thanks to its marvelous healing ability.

Miso Myths

SODIUM

Some people have heard that miso is high in sodium, and therefore, anyone suffering from heart disease or high blood pressure should avoid it. I've seen reports to this effect on the Internet as well; however, research shows that miso does not negatively affect blood pressure. Although miso does tend to have a high sodium content, unlike other high-sodium foods, it doesn't have a negative impact on the cardiovascular system. In a study published in the journal *Hypertension Research*, scientists found that adding sodium to animals' diets significantly increased the animals' blood pressure, whereas consuming a high-miso diet did not affect blood pressure at all.[37] Other research published in the *Journal of Toxologic Pathology* confirmed the results, suggesting that miso is a healthy option even for people who are watching their sodium intake.[38]

THE GREAT SOY DEBATE, ROUND 2

Similar to soy yogurt, during the fermentation process phytic acid found in soy loses its ability to function as an antinutrient. After being fermented it no longer blocks the absorption of nutrients like iron. Additionally, the bioavailability of the beneficial compounds known as isoflavones increases, all of which improves the nutritional value, digestibility, and absorbability of the nutrients found in miso, making it an excellent food choice.

Cancer. Regular consumption of miso has been attributed to many health benefits, including preventing radiation injury and preventing or treating lung, liver, breast, and colon cancers. In one study researchers assessed the long-term effects of miso consumption on

Many people claim that tofu is a fermented food replete with live cultures. In most cases that is not true. Having visited tofu manufacturing plants and even made tofu from scratch, I can say with confidence that most tofu is not fermented and does not contain live cultures. Of course, tofu, like other foods, can be fermented, but that requires it to undergo a special fermentation process that is not part of general tofu manufacturing. Unless the tofu you purchase indicates that it has been fermented and contains live cultures, it doesn't.

animals with lung cancer, concluding that dietary supplementation with long-term fermented miso could exert cancer-preventive effects on lung cancers.[39]

Miso consumption has also been shown to reduce the risk of liver tumors in animal studies, suggesting promise for preventing and possibly reversing liver tumors in men.[40]

Although miso consumption may favor males for its protection against liver tumors, that doesn't mean that miso consumption has no health benefits for females. Multiple studies demonstrate that miso consumption reduces the risk of breast cancer in women. Additional research shows that miso inhibits colon, lung, breast, and liver tumors and may protect against radiation injury when eaten prior to radiation exposure.[41]

Of course, you don't need to eat miso just for its healing properties, as it is a delicious food item as well and lends a unique and rich flavor to soups and salad dressings. Keep in mind that, like all probiotic-rich foods, heating miso destroys the probiotics, so eating miso soup that has been heated to a high temperature (like most miso soup served) is not a good way to enjoy the probiotic benefits it offers.

Super-Healing Sauerkraut

···

I was probably only a few years old when I first tasted sauerkraut. Like most people, my first taste also involved a hot dog
and mustard. But I immediately loved its unique sour and tart
flavor. Later in life I began experimenting with many sauerkraut
combinations, including my favorite one, which is made with
cabbage, apples, and juniper berries. I also love garlic and chili
sauerkraut and have included recipes for both of these types in the
Recipe section.

Sauerkraut isn't just for sausages and hot dogs anymore. This
German staple made of fermented cabbage, though other ingredients are often added to it, offers many impressive health benefits in addition to the obvious delicious taste. New and exciting
research demonstrates the many healing properties of eating naturally fermented sauerkraut on a regular basis, including antibacterial properties, anti-Candida (a commonly occurring fungus),
allergy reduction, improving muscle and exercise recovery in athletes, lowering cholesterol and triglycerides, and regulating certain hormones and reducing hormonally linked cancer growth as
well as directly affecting cancer.

Prevent Food Poisoning. Scientists explored the ability of naturally occurring bacteria that form during the fermentation process
that kill *E. coli* bacteria that would otherwise cause food poisoning. They found that within only two to three days of fermentation
E. coli were not detectable in the vegetable ferment. The naturally
present probiotics *L. plantarum* or *L. mesenteroides* in the fermentation fought off *E. coli* until it was no longer present in the
sauerkraut. Although this study shows the benefits of fermentation
for food preservation, it may also demonstrate the potential of
probiotic-rich vegetable pickles and sauerkraut to kill pathogenic

Kraut and Your Hormones

Let's explore the way sauerkraut may regulate hormones, reduce hormonally linked cancer growth, and directly affect cancer by first examining what happens nutritionally when cabbage is fermenting into its alter ego, sauerkraut. Nutritionally, there are many changes that occur in cabbage during its transformation into sauerkraut. During the fermentation process nutrients known as glucosinolates found in cabbage are transformed into isothiocyanates.[42] Isothiocyanates may suppress tumor growth and excessive hormone production and demonstrate protection against cancer.[43]

E. coli infections present in humans. More research is needed to determine the viability of this possible therapeutic application.[44]

Sauerkraut and naturally pickled vegetables don't just show effectiveness against E. coli; research has also found that L. plantarum strains showed antibacterial activity against other disease-causing bacteria, including Salmonella and Shigella. Salmonella can cause food poisoning, and Shigella are similar bacteria that also cause diarrhea, fever, and stomach cramps.[45] The same study showed that not only did the probiotics in the sauerkraut directly demonstrate antibacterial activity; they also helped boost the immune system activity against disease-causing bacteria.[46]

Help for Candida. Some probiotics are even miniature antifungal-manufacturing facilities. Probiotics in sauerkraut produce anti-Candida compounds to kill some species of Candida fungi. Scientists have found that the probiotics actually produced antifungal compounds to kill Candida and concluded that fermented products of cabbage, like sauerkraut, have therapeutic potential against Candida infections.[47] (For more on Candida, see Chapter 2, page 26.)

Kraut Power for Athletes. Whatever your level of activity, you can benefit from the performance-enhancing capabilities of probiotic-rich foods, regardless of whether you're a professional athlete or a weekend warrior. You may want to take note of the power of fermented foods like sauerkraut to enhance your performance. The Division of Sports Medicine at the University of Hawai'i at Manoa in Honolulu reviewed probiotic-rich foods, including sauerkraut, in the research on athletic performance. They found that numerous health benefits were attributable to probiotic-rich foods on athletic performance, including reducing allergic conditions and enhancing recovery from fatigue as well as improving immune function.[48]

Heart Health. As with yogurt and other fermented foods, new research shows the promise of naturally fermented sauerkraut in reducing cholesterol and triglyceride levels. In animal studies a sauerkraut-derived probiotic was found to offer many heart health benefits, including decreased blood cholesterol and triglyceride levels, and significantly increased levels of powerful antioxidants that protect the body against cellular damage from free radicals.[49]

Cancer. Who knew that eating sauerkraut on a regular basis might also help to keep cancer at bay? Research has shown that fermented cabbage could regulate excessive levels of estrogen, therefore reducing the likelihood of developing estrogen-dependent breast cancer.[50]

An International Flavor

Most people are familiar with German sauerkraut, but it isn't the only type of sauerkraut. The Chinese and Taiwanese also have their traditional versions of naturally fermented pickled cabbage. Actually, the Chinese were the "inventors," or "discoverers" at least, of the art of preserving vegetables through the lactic acid fermentation process, which is also sometimes called pickling. They began employing this discovery over 2,200 years ago in 221 BC. They were trying to provide nutritious foods to the builders of the Great Wall of China during the winter months.

By the thirteenth century the Mongolians brought the Chinese "Suan cai," which means "sour vegetable," with them to Eastern Europe, and it then spread throughout Western Europe as well.[51]

And like the German versions of this delicious and nutritious food, the Asian versions, which typically use Chinese cabbage, also offer many health benefits. In animal studies scientists have found that fermented cabbage regulated the immune system and even demonstrated the ability to reduce or prevent allergic reactions, concluding that Taiwanese fermented cabbage offers promise for the treatment of allergic diseases.[52]

Like the probiotics found in German sauerkraut, those found in Chinese cabbage sauerkraut also exhibited the ability to produce antibacterial compounds against harmful disease-causing bacteria. Scientists identified that the probiotic *L. paracasei HD1.7* produced a compound that kills other bacteria, a bacteriocin, which demonstrated antibacterial activities against a broad spectrum of bacteria, some of which included Proteus, Enterobacter, Staphylococcus, Escherichia, Microccus, Pseudomonas, and Salmonella.[53] You may recognize some of these names from other discussions in this book. The antibacterial effects of Chinese sauerkraut may help in treating these illnesses.

Additional research supports beneficial probiotics' ability to destroy harmful bacteria such as Listeria and Staph infections as well as *E. coli* and Salmonella pathogens.[54] Other scientists have found that particular strains from Chinese sauerkraut demonstrated antimicrobial activity against *E. coli* and Shigella bacteria. They also found that the probiotics reduced cholesterol levels in the animals studied, indicating a possible natural treatment option for infectious conditions and heart disease via its cholesterol-lowering effects.[55]

How to Get the Most Healthful Sauerkraut. Unfortunately, most commercially sold sauerkraut doesn't contain any beneficial probiotics. The traditional process of making sauerkraut involves adding a saltwater solution called a "brine" to shredded cabbage and sometimes other fruit or vegetable ingredients. Then it is left to ferment in large vessels called "crocks," during which the cabbage is weighted down to reduce the amount of oxygen that can access the vegetables as they ferment. This also reduces the chance of spoilage from harmful microbes or mold. However, many manufactures of sauerkraut have taken shortcuts to increase their profits. Instead of waiting for natural fermentation to occur, many instead employ an artificial "pickling"-type process using white vinegar, which doesn't contain any probiotics. And those companies that stay true to natural processes still frequently pasteurize their sauerkraut so it can remain on grocery store shelves for longer periods. This pasteurization or heating process during bottling kills any live cultures that are needed for sauerkraut's health benefits.

It's also important to note that most canning and pickling processes don't actually involve live probiotic cultures. These types of processes usually involve heating foods to high temperatures or placing them in vinegar to preserve them, neither of which encourages probiotic cultures to grow. Besides that, probiotic bacteria wouldn't survive the heat during the canning or bottling process. So don't incorrectly purchase "pickles" from your grocery store thinking that you're getting probiotics. Unless they are found in the refrigerator section and indicate "live cultures" or "unpasteurized," it is unlikely that they contain any probiotics at all.

But there are still some good manufacturers of commercial sauerkraut. You'll typically find these bottles in the refrigerator section of your health food or grocery store. They also indicate that they are *not* pasteurized and/or say "raw" on the label. This usually means that they have the live probiotic cultures that offer the health benefits mentioned in this chapter.

The best way to ensure your sauerkraut is full of active, health-promoting cultures is to make your own. Although you may have heard that this is a difficult process, it is actually quite simple. I provide step-by-step directions and a variety of recipes in the Recipe chapter at the back of this book. Be sure to try my favorite type, Apple-Cabbage Kraut, though I sometimes call it Pink Kraut due to its brilliant pink color. It is made from purple and green cabbage as well as apples and kidney-boosting juniper berries. I first created this recipe after my husband, Curtis, and I were hiking in the Rocky Mountains. We came across a mass of juniper bushes that were thick with berries, so we picked a bunch. I was trying to think of ways to incorporate these kidney-boosting berries into our diet and knew that traditional German sauerkraut often contained juniper berries. The resulting flavor combination is incredible. Now we keep a full crock of Apple-Cabbage Kraut on an ongoing basis. It makes an appealing and colorful side dish for almost any meal. Once you've made your own you'll find it is simple to keep a crock full of fermenting cabbage in your home, ready to add to a meal at a moment's notice. And once you've tasted homemade sauerkraut and the many delicious variations that are possible, you'll want to keep a crock full of it in your kitchen or somewhere else in your home.

What Happens During Sauerkraut and Other Vegetable Fermentation?

There are many different types of fermentation techniques, each one with its own processes involved, but here is the general concept of what occurs during fermentation. Microorganisms, largely bacteria and some yeasts, feed on sugars and starches in the food, thereby converting them into lactic acid. This process is referred to as lacto-fermentation. This is one of the most, if not the most, healthful form of fermentation due to the many lactic acid bacteria formed during the process.

Of course, lactic acid is not the only chemical formed during fermentation; gases, ethanol, other acids, and hydrogen peroxide, among other compounds, are also formed. There are also many precursors to other compounds that form at various stages of the process, resulting in an increase in probiotics, enzymes, vitamins, and more active forms of critical nutrients.

The amount of sauerkraut consumed is only one factor in boosting your health through eating sauerkraut. The variety of sauerkraut also plays a role in its effectiveness. According to Yeong Ju, a researcher at the University of Illinois, there are major differences between sauerkrauts sold in the United States and Poland. She says, "The fermentation process can make a big difference in potency." Much of the sauerkraut sold in stores in North America has been pasteurized, which kills the beneficial bacteria and enzymes and reduces other nutrients. In her research Dr. Ju found that female immigrants to America were four to five times more likely to develop cancer than women who stayed in Poland. She adds that "Polish women eat much more cabbage and sauerkraut, which inhibits estrogen, thereby slowing down the development of the cancer."[56]

I've found some excellent probiotic-rich sauerkraut in health food stores in the refrigerator sections. But making your own is the best way to ensure your sauerkraut contains live probiotics.

Pass the Kimchi—The Health Builder Extraordinaire

Koreans have long known the benefits of fermented vegetables, so much so that their national dish is a combination of fermented Napa cabbage, garlic, onions or scallions, ginger, red pepper or chili peppers, and sometimes other flavor additions. Kimchi (or gimchi or kimchee), the delicious blend of these vegetables, is a traditional food of Korea that has been a part of the country's culture since somewhere between the seventh to eleventh centuries BC. Kimchi is typically eaten as an appetizer or side dish but is often made into main dishes that feature the fermented vegetables, including stew, pancake, soup, and fried rice dishes.

According to Sandor Ellix Katz, author of the book *Wild Fermentation: The Flavor, Nutrition, and Craft of Live-Culture Foods*, there are also varieties of sweeter kimchi that use an assortment of fruit, like plums, apples, pears, pineapple, and grapes, along with the traditional spicy seasonings to make a delicious condiment.[57]

Although taste is an obvious reason to enjoy vegetable or fruit kimchi on a regular basis, so are the many health reasons. And thanks to a small but growing body of research pointing to the significant potential benefits of eating probiotic-rich kimchi, you'll want to enjoy it frequently. Scientists have identified a whopping 970 different bacterial strains in kimchi, representing fifteen different species of probiotics, including *Lactobacillus*, Leuconostoc, and Weissella.[58]

According to additional research, the health properties of kimchi include "anti-cancer, anti-obesity, anticonstipation, colorectal health promotion, probiotic properties, cholesterol reduction, fibrolytic effect (a process that prevents blood clots from growing), antioxidative and anti-aging properties, brain health promotion, immune promotion, and skin health promotion."[59] If a drug were ever released that offered so many health benefits, the demand would exceed production. Although there is no drug that confers all these health benefits, kimchi truly adds weight to the adage "food is the best medicine."

Head Off the Flu Virus. One common criticism of Western medicine has been its inability to provide adequate protection against influenza viruses, which seem to affect many people on a fairly frequent basis. We just suffer through the fevers, chills, aches, malaise, and other undesirable symptoms and possibly reach for our vitamin C, Echinacea, elderberries, and other natural remedies. Or those less inclined toward natural remedies may grab the antihistamines, decongestants, and cough remedies, even though none of these drug options actually reduce the duration of the flu.

As you learned in Chapter 3, if you're seeking protection against flu viruses, you might want to turn to probiotics and probiotic-rich foods. Kimchi is one of the probiotic-rich foods you might want to consider, thanks to its proven flu-fighting capacity. Better yet, add kimchi to your next meal and throughout flu season to help keep the viruses at bay. New research has found that the probiotics found in kimchi confer protection against the flu by regulating the body's innate immunity.[60] They concluded that the *L. plantarum DK119* could be developed as a beneficial antiviral remedy.[61]

Additional Health Benefits. In animal studies scientists have found that particular probiotic strains found in kimchi may prevent memory deficit and concluded that kimchi "may be beneficial for dementia." Obviously, more research needs to be conducted, but considering that there are no known side effects other than additional health benefits of eating kimchi, I would consider it a great dietary addition if you are experiencing memory issues or are trying to prevent them.[62]

In addition to the many other health benefits regular kimchi consumption offers, in animal studies it has also been shown to reduce the inflammation and skin lesions linked with dermatitis.[63] If you have high blood pressure and are worried about your sodium intake, simply choose or make low-sodium kimchi or other fermented foods.

Kombucha—Tea for Vitality

Kombucha (pronounced kom-BOO-shuh) is a beverage that is believed to have been made in Russia and China for over two thousand years, although the exact origin is unknown. The bacteria and yeasts that form the kombucha culture form a type of "floating mat" on the surface of the black or green or other type of tea from which it is typically made.

Although there hasn't been a lot of research conducted on the health benefits of kombucha, there is a large body of anecdotal evidence, some of which has been compiled into whole books on the drink. According to the Moscow Central Bacteriological Institute, kombucha tea may help in addressing immune system deficiencies, cancer, diarrhea, indigestion, prostate problems, male and female incontinence, hemorrhoids, PMS, menopausal symptoms, obesity, aging skin, hair loss, graying hair, kidney stones, gallstones, high cholesterol, hardening of the arteries, acne, psoriasis, diabetes, and hypoglycemia.[64] The Institute also says that kombucha contains many nutrients, including vitamins B_1, B_2, B_3, B_6, B_{12}, folic acid, glucuronic acid, hyaluronic acid, chondroitinsulfate, mucoitinsulfuric acid, and others. Although most of these claims have not been studied, recently the Laboratory of Industrial Microbiology and Food Biotechnology at the University of Latvia assessed existing research on the health benefits of kombucha tea and found that it has four main healing properties, including (1) it improves detoxification, (2) it has antioxidant properties that can counter the effects of harmful free radicals in the body, (3) it has energizing effects, and (4) it improves immunity against some diseases. According to their research, consuming kombucha could help prevent a broad spectrum of metabolic and infectious disorders.[65]

Tea for Diabetes. There are many serious symptoms associated with diabetes, so people with diabetes tend to value any natural food that demonstrates effectiveness at reducing those symptoms. One study conducted in India had results that showed kombucha's "significant anti-diabetic potential."[66]

Tea for Wound Treatment. Kombucha has also shown effectiveness in treating wounds. Researchers at the Department of Pathology, Faculty of Veterinary Medicine, Tehran University, in Iran, found that kombucha was slightly more effective than a medical ointment typically used for skin infections linked to burns or wounds. In the study the researchers divided the animals into two groups: in one group nitrofurazone ointment was applied, and in the other group, kombucha. The researchers assessed the healing of wounds and found that kombucha encouraged healing slightly more than the ointment. They also observed more inflammation in the nitrofurazone group than in the kombucha group.[67]

I'm often asked whether fermented foods like kombucha will contribute to yeast infections. The yeasts found in kombucha are not the same type of yeasts that can cause Candida infections, so you can drink kombucha even if you've had or have Candida overgrowth.

If you're purchasing commercial drinks, please note that most have been pasteurized, which means the live cultures are no longer active. Choose only ones that indicate "nonpasteurized" or "live cultures." Also, kombucha is simple to make at home. We keep a large crock full of kombucha and simply bottle it every two weeks and add new sweetened green tea or licorice root tea to it to keep the cultures active. Check out the Recipe section to learn how to make your own; also, the Resources section offers suggestions for sources of kombucha cultures.

Fermenting Your Own Foods

As you've learned, there are many great health benefits of eating fermented foods. Although it is not necessary to make your own at home, I encourage you to do so. Making homemade yogurt, sauerkraut, kimchi, kombucha, and other cultured foods is much easier than you might think, and it is rewarding and empowering to be creating your own delicious and healing foods. Plus, you can control the ingredients, ensuring no harmful additives. You can also feel confident when you see the transformation of the foods from their original state to their fermented state that you have created probiotic-rich foods with live cultures, something that is hard to trust in many commercial products.

In addition to the nutritional and health benefits of fermentation, the process extends the shelf life of foods. It can also save on food expenses because many foods can be fermented when they are "in season" and used during the winter and spring months when these foods tend to be more expensive. But these are not the only reasons to ferment your own foods; here are twelve more:

1. Budget: Many store-bought fermented foods and superfoods are expensive. You can eat healthy on a budget by making some of your own fermented foods. When cabbage is in season you can create a large crock of sauerkraut, for example, for under a few dollars.
2. Convenience: Once made, fermented foods make everyday meals easier. For example, you might not normally eat a wrap

of cabbage, apples, and cashews, but you can put together a delicious and nutritious wrap of Apple-Cabbage Kraut (page 210) and Roasted Red Pepper Soft Cheese (page 201) made from the same ingredients. It makes day-to-day meals quick and simple.

3. Higher Nutrients: You can purchase locally grown foods or grow your own foods and then ferment them while they are at their peak nutritional state. Most produce travels great distances before it is made into fermented foods like sauerkraut, all the while losing precious nutrients.

4. Higher Potency: The fermentation process activates many nutrients, thereby increasing their absorbability or nutritional potency. Consider that glucosinolates in cabbage become more actively absorbed and better cancer-fighting compounds known as isothiocyanates that flourish during fermentation.

5. Live Cultures: Most store-bought "fermented" foods have actually been pasteurized or heated until there are no cultures left. Some products are artificially flavored or thickened to appear as though they were fermented, when they weren't at all. Many of the health benefits of fermented foods come from the activation of live cultures during the fermentation process—cultures that need to remain intact to obtain these health benefits.

6. More Probiotics: The variety of healthy bacterial strains typically increases when you ferment your own foods. There are different beneficial bacteria in different geographical regions, so some of these bacteria can only be obtained from making your own fermented foods. Additionally, many commercially fermented foods contain only a single strain of bacteria. Yogurt is an excellent example: most commercial varieties contain either a single strain of bacteria or no live cultures at all.

7. Ease: They are easier than you think. Once you've made some of the recipes in *The Probiotic Promise* a few times you'll realize just

how easy it is. It may seem daunting at first because it is learning a new skill and a new way of doing things, but it is remarkably easy once you get used to it.

8. Variety: There are usually only a few types of fermented foods available in most health food stores and fewer still in many grocery stores, but the options for your own homemade ferments are limited only by your imagination. Try some of the recipes at the back of this book first to become accustomed to the techniques, and then have fun experimenting with whatever foods you have on hand or are coming up fresh from your garden.

9. No Waste: Forget throwing out spoiled produce ever again. Simply ferment some of your favorite fruits and veggies, and they'll usually last for months longer than fresh produce. After all, fermentation was originally developed as a simple way to preserve food long before refrigerators were ever invented.

10. Produce Year-Round: In the winter months, when much of the produce sold in grocery stores is flavorless and bland, not to mention nutritionally inferior, enjoy fresh produce that has been fermented. Most fermented foods are packed with the flavors from the produce, any additional spices, as well as the flavor enhancement that results when probiotics work their magic.

11. Better for the Planet: Most "superfoods" travel thousands of miles before you eat them, causing them to have serious environmental implications. Eating more foods that you ferment yourself reduces your ecological footprint.

12. Overall Health: Once you've become accustomed to the various fermentation processes and have made some veggie krauts, dairy-free cheeses, or other delicious treats, you are sure to feel more self-sufficient at using food to maintain or restore your health and the health of your family.

In the next chapter I've provided step-by-step instructions for making the foods discussed in this chapter and many other probiotic-rich foods. Once you've tried many of them you'll definitely want to keep a steady supply of fermented foods as part of your regular diet.

Chapter 7

Easy, Delicious, Probiotic-Rich Recipes

"The time has come to reclaim the stolen harvest
and celebrate the growing and giving of good food
as the highest gift and the most revolutionary act."

—Vandana Shiva, activist

Making your own fermented foods to boost your health and that of your family members is so much easier than you might think. Unlike many store-bought foods that have been pasteurized to kill all the beneficial microbes and enzymes and to destroy various nutrients, the ones you make at home in your kitchen keep all the beneficial microbes intact. In the process of culturing foods to make dairy-free yogurt, cheeses, beverages, breads, sauerkrauts, and other fermented vegetables, you elevate a healthy food into a superfood that has the power to prevent and even eliminate many illnesses.

This chapter includes many of my favorite fermented food recipes so you can make your own delicious, naturally fermented foods such as Dairy-Free Yogurt, Strawberries 'N' Cream Smoothie, Cultured Coconut Milk, Fermented Green Tea

(Kombucha), Roasted Red Pepper Soft Cheese, Apple-Cabbage Kraut, Cultured Anise Carrots, Vanilla Coconut Ice Cream, and Black and Blue Berry Gelato. These foods help you to save money, extend the shelf life of your food, and take your health into your own hands.

Dairy- and Gluten-Free Recipes

All of the recipes are dairy-free and gluten-free so that a greater number of people can enjoy them without suffering ill effects. Many people suffer allergies or sensitivities to these ingredients even without being aware. Most people think that food sensitivities or allergies show up with the same symptoms as seasonal allergies or, in more serious cases, as anaphylactic shock. Although everyone is different and that means a wide variety of symptoms is possible, most people are more likely to suffer bloating, indigestion, nasal congestion, respiratory infections, and ear infections linked to dairy or gluten. In my experience these foods can even aggravate autoimmune disorders sometimes a day or two after eating them, making it extremely difficult to pinpoint the food culprit. To help you boost or restore your health, I steered clear of these ingredients in the recipes below. Even the yogurt and cheese recipes are dairy-free. But don't assume that means they aren't as delicious and creamy as their dairy counterparts— they are. And unlike dairy cheeses, my cheese recipes below are packed with beneficial bacteria to help your health.

Equipment

....

F orget spending a fortune on equipment and ingredients; most of these foods are easy to make with the most basic of kitchen tools and food items. There are a few recipes that would benefit from a crock or large bowl or a special jar for making cultured foods. I've tried to indicate when this is necessary at the beginning of the recipe so you won't get partway through and realize you need something you don't have. But a little resourcefulness can help to keep the costs down. I obtained some of my best fermenting tools from flea markets and garage sales at a fraction of the retail price. I've also provided suppliers in the Resources section so you'll find it easier to track down any recommended special tools.

In the yogurt recipes you may notice that the instructions are for using simple, readily available bowls and other basic kitchen equipment. If you prefer to use a yogurt maker instead, I have recommended one that I like in the Resources section of this book, but it isn't necessary to buy this device. I really like the VitaClay product because the yogurt is made in a clay pot rather than plastic, which can contaminate the yogurt with hormone-disrupting bisphenol-A (BPA) or other toxins found in plastic. Check out my website, www.TheProbioticPromise.com, for more information.

Ingredients

....

Fruits and Vegetables. Most of the recipes call for readily available foods and food ingredients available at your local health food store or market. Of course, if you're growing your own vegetables, you can quickly and easily turn them into probiotic-rich health foods. Many of the fermented vegetable dishes call for cabbage. You can use either green or purple cabbage, depending on your preference. Keep in mind that the taste is quite different after culturing vegetables, so even ones you may not like much could become some of your favorite fermented foods. Cabbage is an excellent example: many people aren't that fond of raw or cooked cabbage but love its transformation into sauerkraut.

You may notice that some vegetables and fruits have a white substance on the outer leaves or skin. This is actually a natural bloom of beneficial microorganisms that also help to encourage the fermentation process when these fruits or vegetables are used. Some of the foods that contain this bloom include apples, blueberries, cabbage, grapes, juniper berries, and plums. When using any of these fruits and vegetables in your fermented foods, wash them but don't wash or wipe off all of this bloom, as it will help to encourage the culturing process.

Some recipes call for "green powder." There are many varieties available. Be sure to choose one that is free of sweeteners, fillers, and gluten. If it doesn't say "gluten-free" on the label, it probably isn't. Some of my preferred choices include chlorella powder or spirulina powder.

Nuts. Many of the yogurt and cheese recipes call for raw, unsalted cashews and almonds, which are available at most health food stores. I've also included suppliers of these foods in the Resources section at the back of this book. These suppliers tend to have superior bulk pricing, which makes using these nuts more affordable. And buying them in bulk tends to make enjoying these foods on a regular basis much more affordable than you'd think.

Salt. You'll notice that many of the recipes call for salt or a "brine," which is simply a saltwater solution. Choose unrefined sea salt or Himalayan pink salt wherever possible, as it contains trace amounts of beneficial nutrients your body needs for health.

The media and many nutritionists seem to be telling people that the amount of nutrient variation between unrefined sea salt and table salt is negligible and doesn't make a difference to health, but this is incorrect. Our bodies need many trace minerals. Note the word "trace," which indicates the minute amounts needed, but they are still essential building blocks of our bodies' cells and tissues. Avoid using table salt, or iodized salt as it is also called, because it can interfere with the natural fermentation process. The iodine it contains is an antimicrobial mineral that can block the growth of probiotic bacteria cultures. If you use coarse, unrefined sea salt, double the amount of salt when a recipe calls for fine, unrefined sea salt or just indicates unrefined sea salt.

Sweeteners. When the recipes call for one of these natural sweeteners, do not substitute artificial sweeteners or the natural sweetener stevia. The probiotic cultures need sugar molecules to feed on in order to proliferate. Artificial sweeteners are not food, should never be consumed by humans, and have been linked to a list of over one hundred health conditions. See my book *Weekend Wonder Detox* for more information. In addition to the many health problems artificial sweeteners cause for humans, probiotics do not recognize them as food.

The herb stevia is a great natural sweetener for human use, but because it just naturally tastes sweet and doesn't actually contain any sugar molecules, the probiotics can't use it as food to proliferate.

Occasionally, you may see a recipe that calls for D-ribose as an optional sweetener. D-ribose is a natural sweetener that is tremendously healing for the body. Research shows that the body metabolizes D-ribose to create adenosine triphosphate (ATP), which is the body's energy supply and is used by every cell for every metabolic function. D-ribose helps by resetting the body's ATP levels, thereby supplying the body with sufficient energy for burning fat, balancing blood sugar levels, warding off cravings, boosting energy levels, and improving heart and muscle function. Many athletes also take D-ribose to boost endurance levels, performance, and recovery time. It is a valuable aid to chronic fatigue syndrome and fibromyalgia sufferers. Because it can be expensive, any recipes that use D-ribose call for small amounts simply to boost up the health benefits of the food. If you would rather use another natural sweetener like honey, agave nectar, pure maple syrup (not the pancake syrup most people use), or coconut sugar, that is fine.

Whey. There are many different ways to ferment foods, including in whey, in brine, in vinegar, and through the addition of probiotic powder, to name a few. Whey is the clearish-yellowish liquid that is normally strained off when dairy or dairy-free milk is made into yogurt. During the yogurt-making process the dairy or dairy-free milk separates into two parts: the thick, creamy part that constitutes the yogurt and the remaining liquid part called whey. This normally discarded substance can be saved and used for easy pickling of many different fruits and vegetables, as a starter for a new batch of yogurt, or as an addition to smoothies for an instant probiotic boost.

Yogurt

Dairy-Free Yogurt

Servings: 8 (approximately ¾ cup each)

I encourage you to make Dairy-Free Yogurt as one of the first recipes you start with. During the fermentation process the almond or soy milk separates into yogurt and whey. The yogurt is the thicker, creamy, white portion, and the whey is the clearish-yellowish liquid that you strain off. Most people who make yogurt simply throw away the whey, yet it is full of active cultures that can be used to make countless other cultured creations. Save the whey in a glass jar in the refrigerator so you can make various recipes that follow.

Notes about ingredients: Be sure to choose only organic soy milk because soy is a heavily genetically modified crop.

For the sweetener, remember that stevia won't work, as the cultures need the sugar to feed on.

See Chapter 5 and the Resources section for information on finding a high-quality probiotic powder.

1 1.8-quart or -liter package of almond or organic soy milk

2 tablespoons raw, unpasteurized honey or agave or other natural sweetener

3 capsules of your favorite probiotic powder or 1 teaspoon of powdered probiotics

In a medium-sized saucepan over low to medium heat, heat the almond or soy milk until it is just slightly warm. Dissolve the honey or agave, and remove from the heat. Empty the contents of the probiotic capsules or add the probiotic powder to the almond or soy milk, and stir until combined. Never add probiotic powder to hot almond or soy milk, as it will kill the active cultures. If the milk is too hot (above 115 degrees Fahrenheit), simply wait until it has cooled to a lukewarm (100 to 115 degrees Fahrenheit) temperature.

Pour the milk into a glass or ceramic bowl. Cover with a clean tea towel, and let sit in a warm—but not hot—place where it will remain undisturbed for at least 8 hours. Ideally, the inside of an oven with the pilot light (but not the heat) on is perfect. Allow to sit for at least 8 hours, undisturbed. If you prefer a tangier yogurt, leave for 10 hours. Gently remove the bowl from the oven.

Scoop out the thick yogurt and place in a bowl with a lid, preferably a glass bowl. Do not use metal, as metal can damage the cultures. Reserve the remaining clearish-yellowish liquid—the whey—as it can be used in many recipes that follow. You can also add the whey to juices or smoothies for a quick probiotic boost. Store the yogurt in the refrigerator, where it will last for about 2 weeks. In a separate glass container, store the whey in the refrigerator. It will also last about 2 weeks.

Dairy-Free Whey

Servings: 8 (approximately ¼ cup each)
Follow all instructions for Dairy-Free Yogurt. Scoop off the thick yogurt after it has cultured, and pour the remaining clearish-yellowish liquid—the whey—through a cheesecloth-lined sieve. Store the filtered liquid in the refrigerator in a glass jar or container for up to two weeks. This is the whey that you will use for many of the recipes throughout this book. You can add a quarter to half cup to a smoothie recipe, use half a cup of whey to start your next batch of yogurt, or add it to a saltwater solution (brine) to expedite the growth of probiotics in various vegetables, including onions, beans, grated carrots, ground chilies, cucumbers, or any others you might like to try. When using whey to ferment vegetables, simply follow the instructions outlined with one of the vegetable recipes below. Keeping whey on hand in the fridge is an easy way to get more probiotic-rich foods into your diet and to simplify the process of making fermented foods.

Savory Dairy-Free Greek-Style Yogurt

Servings: 8 (approximately ⅔ cup each)
Like the Dairy-Free Yogurt above, this is a good recipe to start with. The fermentation process causes the almond-cashew-sunflower mixture to separate into yogurt and whey. The yogurt is the thicker, creamy, white portion, and the whey is the clearish-yellowish liquid that you strain off. In this case,

because of the specific nuts and seeds I chose to make it, the resulting yogurt turned out to be quite thick. Save the whey in a glass jar in the refrigerator so you can make many of the cultured creations that follow. The thicker Greek-style yogurt is perfect for making tzatziki, a delicious Greek dip for vegetables, pita bread, or bread, or just enjoying as a quick and easy breakfast. If it starts to turn a light grayish color, don't worry—it is normal. The sunflower seeds in the recipe cause this to happen.

See Chapter 5 and the Resources for information on finding a high-quality probiotic powder.

For the sweetener, remember that stevia won't work, as the cultures need the sugar to feed on.

- -

½ cup raw, unsalted almonds

½ cup raw, unsalted cashews

½ cup raw, unsalted sunflower seeds

2 tablespoons raw, unpasteurized honey or agave or other natural sweetener

4 cups filtered, unchlorinated water

2 capsules of your favorite probiotic powder or 1 teaspoon powdered probiotics

- -

In a high-powered blender, blend the almonds, cashews, sunflower seeds, honey, and water until smooth. In a medium-sized saucepan over low to medium heat, heat the nut-seed-honey milk until it is just slightly warm, then remove from the heat. Empty the contents of the probiotic capsules or add the probiotic powder to the almond-cashew-sunflower seed milk and stir until combined.

Pour the milk into a glass or ceramic bowl. Cover with a clean tea towel, and let sit in a warm but not hot (100 to 115 degrees Fahrenheit) place, where it will remain undisturbed for at least 8 hours. Ideally, the inside of an oven with the pilot light (but not the heat) on is perfect. Allow to sit for at least 8 hours, undisturbed. If you prefer a tangier yogurt, leave for 10 hours. Gently remove the bowl from the oven.

Scoop out the thick yogurt and place in a bowl with a lid, preferably a glass bowl. Do not use metal, as metal can damage the cultures. Reserve the remaining clearish-yellowish liquid—the whey—as it can be used in many recipes that follow. You can also add the whey to juices or smoothies for a quick probiotic boost. Store the yogurt in the refrigerator, where it will last for about 2 weeks. In a separate glass container, store the whey in the refrigerator; it will also last about 2 weeks.

Savory Greek-Style Yogurt (Made with Whey)

Servings: 8 (approximately ¾ cup each)

The following recipe is similar to Dairy-Free Greek-Style Yogurt but is made in a slightly different manner. Use the previous recipe if you don't have any whey on hand; use this one if you have whey that you'd like to use. Using whey as a starter can help you save money on probiotic powder.

½ cup raw, unsalted almonds

½ cup raw, unsalted cashews

½ cup raw, unsalted sunflower seeds

2 tablespoons raw, unpasteurized honey or agave or other natural sweetener (*note*: stevia won't work, as the cultures need the sugar to feed on)

4 cups filtered, unchlorinated water

¼ cup whey (the clearish-yellowish liquid left over from making yogurt)

In a high-powered blender, blend the almonds, cashews, sunflower seeds, honey, and water. Pour the milk into a glass or ceramic bowl, and stir in the whey until it is combined. Cover with a clean tea towel, and let sit in a warm but not hot (100 to 115 degrees Fahrenheit) place where it will remain undisturbed for 6 to 8 hours. Ideally, the inside of an oven with the pilot light (but not the heat) on is perfect. Allow to sit for at least 8 hours, undisturbed. If you prefer a tangier yogurt, leave for 10 hours. Gently remove the bowl from the oven.

Scoop out the thick yogurt, and place in a bowl with a lid, preferably a glass bowl. Do not use metal, as metal can damage the cultures. Reserve the remaining clearish-yellowish liquid—the whey—as it can be used in many recipes that follow. You can also add the whey to juices or smoothies for a quick probiotic boost. Store the yogurt in the refrigerator, where it will last for about 2 weeks. In a separate glass container, store the whey in the refrigerator; it will also last about 2 weeks.

Sweet Yogurt

Servings: 8 (approximately ⅔ cup each)

The following recipe is similar to the other yogurt recipes, but you'll use yogurt from a previous batch or store-bought yogurt with live cultures as the starter for this recipe. By simply saving a half cup of yogurt from each batch and using it to make a new batch of yogurt, you can keep your probiotic cultures alive indefinitely. I make this recipe once or twice a week, always reserving a half cup of yogurt for the next batch. Doing so also saves you money. If you don't have any yogurt on hand, substitute one-half cup of whey. If you don't have any whey on hand, use three capsules of probiotics, emptied into the liquid, instead. This yogurt is sweeter-tasting than the savory options, making it a great choice when you want yogurt for breakfast or for sweet dishes or desserts. It's my favorite one, so I keep it going on a regular basis to enjoy with seasonal fruit for breakfast. It is great served with fresh blueberries, peaches, or strawberries or topped with raw, unsalted walnuts and a drizzle of honey for a delicious Greek-inspired dessert.

Notes on ingredients: For the sweetener, remember that stevia won't work, as the cultures need the sugar to feed on.

½ cup raw, unsalted almonds

½ cup raw, unsalted cashews

2 tablespoons raw, unpasteurized honey or agave or other natural sweetener

4 cups filtered, unchlorinated water

½ cup yogurt (you can use store-bought yogurt or, once you've made this recipe just save ½ cup to make the next batch of yogurt) or ½ teaspoon probiotic powder, or 2 capsules of probiotics, contents emptied

In a high-powered blender, blend the almonds, cashews, honey, water, and yogurt. Pour the almond-cashew milk into a glass or ceramic bowl or a yogurt maker. Cover with a clean tea towel, and let sit in a warm but not hot (100 to 115 degrees Fahrenheit) place where it will remain undisturbed for 6 to 8 hours. If you're using a yogurt maker, follow the manufacturer's directions. Ideally, the inside of an oven with the pilot light (but not the heat) on is fine. Allow to sit for at least 6 hours, undisturbed. If you prefer a tangier yogurt, leave for 10 hours. Gently remove the bowl from the oven or yogurt maker.

Scoop out the thick yogurt and place in a bowl with a lid, preferably a glass bowl. Do not use metal, as metal can damage the cultures. Reserve the remaining clearish-yellowish liquid—the whey—as it can be used in many recipes that follow. You can also add the whey to juices or smoothies for a quick probiotic boost. Store the yogurt in the refrigerator, where it will last for about 2 weeks. In a separate glass container, store the whey in the refrigerator; it will also last about 2 weeks.

Beverages

Blueberry Banana Smoothie

Servings: 2 (approximately 1¾ cups each)

This delicious blueberry smoothie is packed with probiotics (as long as you use a yogurt that contains live cultures) and proanthocyanidins. Proanthocyanidins are a type of naturally occurring plant chemical that has been shown to aid allergies, improve brain health and memory, contain anticancer properties, and help heal heart disease. You'll love the taste as much as the health benefits of this smoothie that makes a great breakfast, snack, or healthy dessert.

> 1 cup Sweet Yogurt (see page 191, or other type of your favorite yogurt)
>
> 1 cup filtered, unchlorinated water or almond milk
>
> 1 cup frozen blueberries
>
> ½ frozen banana

Blend all ingredients together until smooth. Enjoy immediately!

Curtis's Chocolate Banana Pro Smoothie

Servings: 2 (approximately 1⅔ cups each)

My husband, Curtis, created this delicious smoothie for those times when he wanted all of the nutritional and probiotic benefits of a smoothie while still feeling like he is having a decadent chocolate milkshake. Because it is packed with nutritional goodness, it makes a great breakfast, snack, postworkout replenishment, or dessert. The addition of chia seeds adds fiber and essential fatty acids, while hemp protein powder or pumpkin-seed protein powder are excellent sources of protein.

- 1 cup almond yogurt (see Savory Dairy-Free Greek-Style Yogurt recipe, page 188)

- 1 cup almond milk

- 1 frozen banana

- 1 tablespoon cocoa powder (more if you desire a "chocolate-ier" taste)

- 1 tablespoon chia seeds (optional)

- 1 tablespoon green powder (optional)

- 1 tablespoon hemp or pumpkin-seed protein powder (or other protein powder of your choice)

Blend all ingredients together until smooth. Enjoy immediately!

Strawberries 'N' Cream Smoothie

Servings: 2 (approximately 2 cups each)

Strawberries are antioxidant powerhouses that fight aging and disease—only eight strawberries contain more vitamin C than an orange. They have been shown to help prevent heart disease, arthritis, memory loss, and cancer. This smoothie offers all the nutritional benefits of strawberries with the healing properties of probiotics, provided you use a yogurt rich in live cultures. I encourage you to make the Sweet Yogurt ahead of time and keep it on hand for quick and delicious smoothies like this one. It's so good you'll forget it is healthy.

- 1 cup Sweet Yogurt (see page 191, or use your favorite yogurt)

- 1 cup almond milk

- 1 frozen banana

- 1 cup frozen strawberries

Blend all ingredients together until smooth. Enjoy immediately!

Cultured Coconut Milk

Yield: approximately 1 quart/liter

This "milk" is a naturally sweet and delicious alternative to dairy milk, plus it contains health-promoting medium-chain triglycerides (MCTs) that rev metabolism and help to reset the thyroid gland, a butterfly-shaped gland in the throat that regulates metabolism and body temperature. It is simple to make and great to keep on hand to drink on its own, add to smoothies, or to make the delicious Coconut Ice Cream recipe below.

1 cup unsweetened dried coconut

4 cups filtered, unchlorinated water

1 tablespoon raw, unpasteurized honey or agave nectar

½ cup whey or 2 probiotic capsules

Blend the coconut, water, and honey together until smooth. Pour into a large glass or ceramic bowl or a yogurt maker. Add the whey or the contents of the probiotic capsules, and stir to combine. Cover with a cloth or the lid to the yogurt maker. Let rest in a warm location where it will be undisturbed for 8 hours. Pour through a sieve and into a glass bottle or pitcher. Refrigerate. Lasts about 1 week in the refrigerator.

Fermented Green Tea (Kombucha)

It may seem a bit intimidating to brew a fermented tea whose name you might not even have known about prior to reading *The Probiotic Promise*. I too was quite uncertain about it when I brewed and fermented my first batch of kombucha, but I soon discovered that it is simple to do.

You'll need to obtain a kombucha culture, which looks like an oddly colored, somewhat flat cap that forms on the top of the kombucha. See the Resources section for places to obtain kombucha cultures. Don't be alarmed about the amount of sugar in the recipe; it is the food for the kombucha culture and allows it to grow. Without the sugar it won't work. And, sorry, stevia won't work either, as it doesn't contain any sugar molecules. During the fermentation process the sugar is transformed into the beneficial probiotics and other nutritional constituents that make kombucha so health promoting. After five days to a week of fermentation there is almost no sugar left.

When making kombucha it is important to make sure your hands are clean. Identify an undisturbed part of your kitchen where your kombucha can ferment away from drafts, sunlight, people, and animals.

MATERIALS AND INGREDIENTS

Ceramic crock or wide-mouthed glass water jug, preferably with a spigot or tap on it

4 quarts/liters filtered, unchlorinated water

1 cup sugar

4 to 6 green or black tea bags or 4 teaspoons loose-leaf tea

1 piece of clean linen or cotton big enough to cover the crock or glass jug. Cheesecloth is too porous, so it is best avoided. Also, avoid synthetic fabrics.

1 large stainless steel pot

1 wooden spoon

1 elastic band or string to secure the linen over the top of the crock

Making Your Kombucha

You can use any wide-mouthed vessel, bowl, or crock. I use a crock with a spigot on the side for one batch of kombucha and an inexpensive glass water jug with a spigot for another so I can keep two types of kombucha brewing at the same time. You can use either of these types of vessels for your kombucha. Make sure the vessel is thoroughly cleaned prior to use. You can mist it with 3 percent food-grade hydrogen peroxide to sterilize it before using so as to help ensure it is free of harmful microbes. Rinse it out afterward.

Bring the water to a boil, add the sugar, and stir until dissolved. Then add the green or black tea bags, and boil for an additional few minutes. Then turn off the heat and allow to steep for 15 minutes. Although some people claim tea should not be boiled, it is an essential part of the kombucha process to help kill any mold spores growing on the tea leaves. Remove the tea bags. Allow the tea to cool to room temperature or slightly lukewarm temperature (70 to 75 degrees Fahrenheit). Any hotter than this can damage the kombucha culture. Pour the steeped tea into the crock or vessel you're using. Add the kombucha mother (starter culture) and the tea it came with to the vessel. Cover the top of the vessel with the cloth, and place the elastic band around the rim to hold the cloth in place. Alternatively, use tape around the edge to hold the cloth in place. This helps to ensure that the cloth won't fall into the crock.

Place the covered crock in a quiet area with air ventilation in a warm but not sunlit area where it will not be disturbed. The ideal fermentation temperature range is 73 to 82 degrees Fahrenheit, or 23 to 28 degrees Celsius. Once you've located a spot for it do not move it while the kombucha is fermenting, as it may interfere with the culturing process.

The kombucha will be ready in about 7 to 10 days, depending on your preference for tartness or sweetness. The longer the brewing time, the more tart the kombucha will be. Shorter times result in a sweeter kombucha (and typically contain more sugar, so if you're trying to avoid sugar, opt for longer brewing times). Don't worry if you smell a slight vinegary aroma; this is normal.

Harvest Your Kombucha Tea

After 7 to 10 days have passed, check the taste of your kombucha. If it is sweeter than you'd like, allow it to ferment another day or two. If it has a vinegary taste, you may need to bottle future batches after a fewer number of days. It is still fine to drink, but it may need to be diluted with water at the time of drinking to avoid irritating your mucus membranes. Remove the cloth from the crock. You'll probably see the large, original culture and a newly formed culture on top. The larger culture is referred to as the "mother" and the smaller culture is called the "baby." You can remove the newly formed baby and store it in a glass jar with two cups of the kombucha tea in the refrigerator as a backup should you need another culture. Alternatively, you can give the "baby" away to a friend or family member to get them started making kombucha.

Pour all but approximately 2 cups of your fermented kombucha tea into a glass jar or container with a lid and store it in the refrigerator. Once every week or so, loosen the lid of the kombucha in the fridge to allow gases to escape. To keep an ongoing supply of kombucha, follow the above instructions to brew additional tea, allow to cool, and add to the remaining 2 cups left in the kombucha fermenting crock. Follow these instructions every week to ten days, and you'll have kombucha on a regular basis. Drink 2 to 4 ounces of kombucha tea 1 to 3 times daily with meals or before meals. Avoid drinking kombucha if you have an ulcer, as the acetic acid that naturally forms during the fermentation process can irritate the ulcer.

There may be times when you don't notice a "baby" culture. That usually is due to the temperature of the room. If the room is too cold, a baby may not form. It is not a concern if this doesn't happen. This may indicate that you may need to add a few days to your fermentation time for the kombucha to develop sufficient probiotic cultures.

If the kombucha culture drops to the bottom of the crock, it means that the temperature of the tea was too hot and has likely destroyed the cultures that ferment kombucha. You'll need to start over with a fresh culture if this happens.

If at any time you see mold on your kombucha culture or a bluish-green growth, throw out both the kombucha culture and the tea. Clean the crock thoroughly, and disinfect with food-grade hydrogen peroxide before preparing another batch. If the entire kombucha turns brown, it may have become contaminated with harmful microorganisms and should not be used.

Dairy-Free Cheese

Creamy Dairy-Free Yogurt Cheese

Yield: approximately 1½ cups, or 8 3-tablespoon servings

1 batch of yogurt from any of the recipes above

½ teaspoon of salt, or to taste

1 teaspoon raw, unpasteurized honey or agave,
or to taste

After separating the thick yogurt from the whey, line the inside of a strainer with a few layers of cheesecloth. (Cheesecloth is available from most health food stores, hardware stores, and grocery stores. See the Resources section for suppliers of unbleached cheesecloth.) Make sure the cheesecloth is large enough to go beyond the edges of the strainer. Scoop the yogurt into the cheesecloth-lined strainer. Allow the yogurt to strain for at least an hour. The liquid that pours off is whey that can be reserved for other recipes that follow. Reserve the strained yogurt, which is now thicker yogurt. Add salt and honey to taste. Stir together until mixed. Serve as a soft yogurt cheese on top of cooked sweet potatoes, spread on crackers or bread, or add some fresh herbs as a dip for vegetables. Lasts approximately 1 week in the refrigerator.

Soft and Creamy Dairy-Free Cheese

Yield: approximately 2 cups, or 10 3-tablespoon servings

No one will guess this is a dairy-free cheese. It's so creamy and delicious, and it actually offers more health benefits than dairy cheese thanks to its unique probiotic-rich fermentation process. It takes about eight to ten hours to ferment but can be whipped up with only ten minutes of preparation time.

. . . .

2 cups raw, unsalted cashews, soaked overnight or for 10 to 12 hours

1 teaspoon probiotic powder or 2 probiotic capsules, opened (check the Resources section at the back of this book for sources), dissolved in 1 cup filtered, unchlorinated water

1 teaspoon unrefined sea salt, or to taste

1 to 2 teaspoons onion powder

¼ teaspoon ground nutmeg

. . . .

In a blender or food processor, combine the drained cashews and the probiotic powder and water mixtures. Blend until smooth. Place in a glass bowl, cover with a clean cloth, and let rest for 10 to 14 hours to ferment. Then stir in the salt, onion powder, and nutmeg until well mixed. Form the cheese into a ball or press it into a springform pan. Serve with crackers, pitas, or vegetable crudités. Lasts about 2 weeks in the refrigerator.

Almond Ricotta Cheese
. . . .
Yield: 1 to 2 cups

This is a delicious dairy-free almond ricotta cheese made by making almond yogurt, thickening it, and adding a couple of flavorings. It is delicious in stuffed pasta, on toast, or as a pasta or dessert topping.

. . . .

1 quart/liter unsweetened almond milk

2 tablespoons plus 1 teaspoon raw, unpasteurized honey or agave nectar

2 capsules probiotics or ½ teaspoon probiotic powder

Dash unrefined sea salt

. . . .

Pour the almond milk into a clean ceramic crock or bowl with a lid. Add 2 tablespoons of honey and stir until combined. Empty the probiotic capsules by removing one end and dumping the contents into the almond milk mixture. Discard the empty capsules. Stir the almond milk until the probiotic powder is incorporated. Cover. Place in a warm, undisturbed place for 8 to 10 hours. The inside of an oven with the pilot light left on is ideal.

Uncover and carefully scoop the thick portion of the resulting almond yogurt into a fine sieve lined with cheesecloth. Place the resulting thickened yogurt in a bowl, and continue until all of the yogurt has been filtered. Save the clearish-yellowish liquid—the whey—for use in other fermented recipes.

Add the remaining 1 teaspoon honey and sea salt to the thickened yogurt. Use as you would ricotta cheese. Lasts about 1 week in the refrigerator.

Roasted Red Pepper Soft Cheese

Yield: approximately 2 cups, or 10 3-tablespoon servings

This soft cheese makes the perfect cheese to serve with crackers, pita wedges, or with vegetable crudités. It has a rich flavor and texture, making it suitable to make into a cheese ball, log, or to serve as a dip. The fermentation process increases the number of probiotics, making it a delicious and healthy way to improve the bacterial balance in your body.

1 cup raw, unsalted cashews

1 cup filtered, unchlorinated water

1 capsule or ½ teaspoon probiotic powder

1 tablespoon coconut oil or extra virgin olive oil

½ small onion, minced

½ red pepper, finely chopped

½ teaspoon unrefined sea salt

Soak the cashews in water for 4 hours or overnight; blend together. Add the probiotics; stir together until mixed. Cover with a clean cloth, and let sit for 8 to 10 hours in a warm, undisturbed location.

In a medium pan over low to medium heat, sauté the onion and red pepper in oil until soft and lightly caramelized, about 15 minutes. Allow to cool. Add the onion–red pepper mixture and salt to the cashews, and stir together until mixed.

Form the cheese into a ball or press into a small spring-form pan. Serve with crackers, pita wedges, or vegetable crudités. Spread on sandwiches or add to wraps. Thin with a little water for a delicious salad dressing. Lasts about 1 week in the refrigerator.

Cashew-Thyme Soft Cheese

Yield: approximately 2 cups, or 10 3-tablespoon servings

Rich in omega-3 fatty acids, cashews impart a delicious flavor and creamy texture to this soft cheese. I serve this cheese during the holiday season because the flavors seem to fit perfectly with the holidays. Unlike most holiday food, it doesn't come with the guilt. It's packed with health-building probiotics that increase during the fermentation process.

1 cup raw, unsalted cashews

1 cup filtered, unchlorinated water

1 capsule or ½ teaspoon probiotic powder

1 tablespoon coconut oil or extra virgin olive oil

½ small onion, minced

1 spring fresh thyme, with stems removed

½ teaspoon unrefined sea salt

Soak the cashews in water for 4 hours or overnight; blend together. Add the probiotics; stir together until mixed. Cover with a clean cloth, and let sit for 8 to 10 hours in a warm, undisturbed location.

In a medium pan over low to medium heat, sauté the onion and thyme in oil until soft and lightly caramelized, about 15 minutes. Allow to cool. Add the onion-thyme mixture and salt to the cashews, and stir together until mixed.

Form the cheese into a bowl or press into a small springform pan. Serve with crackers, pita wedges, or vegetable crudités. Spread on sandwiches or add to wraps. Thin with a little water for a delicious salad dressing. Lasts about 1 week in the refrigerator.

Basil–Pumpkin Seed Soft Cheese

Yield: approximately 1½ cups, or 12 2-tablespoon servings

This soft cheese has all the flavor of fresh basil combined with the many health benefits of pumpkin seeds that are rich in omega-3 fatty acids. Omega-3s are naturally anti-inflammatory, helping to keep pain levels down and metabolism up.

1 cup raw, unsalted pumpkin seeds

Water, filtered and unchlorinated, just enough to cover

1 capsule or ¼ teaspoon probiotic powder

1 teaspoon extra virgin olive oil

2 tablespoons minced onions

1 handful fresh basil, about 8 to 10 leaves

Dash sea salt, or to taste

Place the pumpkin seeds in a small glass or ceramic bowl, and cover with just enough water to submerge the seeds. Cover with a lid or clean cloth, and leave for 4 to 8 hours, or overnight.

Puree the pumpkin seeds with enough water to create a soft cheese consistency and to allow the seeds to grind into a smooth texture.

Place the mixture back into the glass or ceramic bowl. Add the contents of the probiotic capsule by removing one end, or add the probiotic powder; stir to mix. Cover with a lid or clean cloth, and let sit for 8 to 10 hours or until the desired taste has been reached.

In a small frying pan, heat the oil over low to medium heat, then add the minced onion. Sauté until the onions have lightly caramelized, about 15 minutes. Do not allow the oil to smoke. Allow onions to cool.

Meanwhile, finely mince the basil, and add to the pumpkin seed–probiotic mixture. Add the caramelized onion and a dash of salt, or to taste. Mix together and form desired shape, such as a log, cheeseball, or simply place in a bowl as a dip. Serve.

Keeps for about a week covered and refrigerated.

Mild Cheese

Yield: approximately 1½ cups, or 12 2-tablespoon servings

This is my favorite probiotic-rich, dairy-free cheese. It is super-creamy, sliceable, and even melts well, although I don't recommend heating it, as you'll destroy the beneficial cultures. The cheese can be enjoyed on its own or with crackers and fresh bread.

1 cup raw, unsalted cashews

1 cup filtered, unchlorinated water

1 capsule probiotics or ½ teaspoon probiotic powder

⅓ cup coconut oil, melted but not hot

1 tablespoon dark brown miso

⅓ teaspoon sea salt

Soak cashews in water for 8 hours or overnight. Blend together with just enough of the soak water to create a smooth texture. Pour into a glass or ceramic bowl. Empty the contents of the probiotic capsule or add the probiotic powder; stir together. Cover with a cloth, and allow to ferment for 8 to 12 hours, depending on taste preference (shorter fermentation times create a milder cheese, whereas longer times develop a stronger cheese flavor).

Blend all the ingredients together. Pour into a small glass bowl lined with cheesecloth, smoothing out air pockets. Allow to chill in the refrigerator until firm, or at least 2 hours. Remove from the fridge. Remove the cheese from the bowl, and remove the cheesecloth. Serve.

Serving options: Serve on its own or with balsamic vinegar, fresh fruit, or cranberry chutney. Lasts about 2 weeks in the refrigerator.

Salad Dressings

Dairy-Free, Probiotic-Rich Caesar Salad Dressing

Yield: approximately 2 cups

No one will know that this delicious Caesar salad dressing is dairy-free. It is thick and creamy and tastes amazing. You can toss it with Romaine lettuce for a quick and tasty salad, but you can also use it as a vegetable or bread dip.

2 cups Savory Greek-Style Yogurt

1 lemon, juiced

Dash cayenne

¼ teaspoon unrefined sea salt

1 small garlic clove

Blend all ingredients together until smooth. Store in a covered jar in the fridge for up to 1 week.

Ginger Vinaigrette

Servings: 8 (approximately 2 tablespoons each)

This delicious vinaigrette offers the natural probiotics found in miso. It has a delicate yet slightly spicy flavor thanks to the heat from the fresh ginger. It's perfect on a bed of greens, on mung bean sprouts, or over a slaw-style salad of grated vegetables.

⅔ cup extra virgin olive oil

⅓ cup rice wine vinegar

2 tablespoons dark brown miso

1 teaspoon raw, unpasteurized honey or other natural sweetener

1 tablespoon fresh ginger, grated

Combine all ingredients in a jar or blender, and shake or blend together until well mixed. Refrigerate unused portions for up to 1 month.

Green Tea–Lime Vinaigrette/Marinade

Yield: approximately 1⅔ cups

I was slow at bottling a batch of green tea kombucha, so it turned a bit "vinegar-y." I decided to try it as a marinade for vegetables, salmon, and beans, all of which turned out quite tasty. You obtain the many health benefits of green tea, including protection against the sun's harmful UV rays, cancer, heart disease, fat burning, blood sugar balancing, and even wrinkle prevention, thanks to its naturally occurring compound called epigallocatechin gallate (EGCG).

1 cup green tea kombucha

½ cup olive oil

1 teaspoon unrefined sea salt

1 1-inch piece of ginger, grated

1 lime, juiced, plus zest of ½ lime

2 teaspoons coconut sugar or 1 teaspoon raw,
    unpasteurized honey

. . . .

Combine all ingredients in a jar or blender, and shake or blend
together. Refrigerate unused portions for up to 1 month.

Veggie Ferments

My grandfather was born in Austria and came to Canada
when he was a small boy. He came with his mother, sister, and a tradition of fermented foods that he later taught to my
grandmother, who kept the sauerkraut tradition alive in my family. I am happy to share the recipe for a simple sauerkraut along
with others I developed to enjoy a wide range of sauerkraut flavors.

I've found a great product called the Probiotic Jar that makes
fermenting vegetables, sauerkraut, dill pickles, and just about anything else almost completely foolproof. It involves a special "air
lock" that pulls any remaining oxygen out of the glass jar that
contains the food awaiting fermentation. Because the microbes
involved in food spoilage require oxygen to thrive and the probiotic bacteria that ferment foods and improve our health do not
need oxygen, this process almost guarantees great results without the spoilage or worry. According to research by the manufacturer of the Probiotic Jar, beneficial bacteria double their numbers
every twenty to thirty minutes until they run out of carbohydrates to consume, which translates into more beneficial bacteria
for you. And for those of you wondering, it is made of lead-free
glass, so you don't have to worry about heavy metals or harmful

toxins like BPA in plastic—it doesn't contain them. Check out the Resources section of this book for more information about this handy invention.

Simple Sauerkraut

Servings: 20 (approximately 1 cup each)

This sauerkraut is a "plain" sauerkraut without the many possible flavor additions. It is delicious on its own, but feel free to add a handful of flavor additions if you prefer. Some possibilities include caraway seeds, fennel seeds, coriander seeds, juniper berries, fresh basil, fresh or dried rosemary, mustard seeds, or others. Use your imagination if you want to try different flavors of sauerkraut, but feel free to also enjoy this simple sauerkraut recipe "as is," because it has a great flavor all on its own.

Making homemade sauerkraut or other type of vegetable "sauerkraut" is easier than you might think. In addition to being packed with health-building probiotics that are usually deficient in store-bought kraut, homemade kraut tastes so much better. The technique description below may seem intensive, but once you get used to the basic process, it's actually simple.

You can use a variety of fermentation vessels, ranging from small to large stoneware crocks, ceramic or glass bowls, to wide-mouthed mason jars. Avoid using metal or plastic containers, as the level of acidity will increase, which can cause a chemical reaction with the metal or plastic. Additionally, most beneficial microbes do not grow well in a metal container. Glass, ceramic, or stoneware is best.

Whatever type you use, you'll need a plate, jar, or cover that fits inside the crock, bowl, or jar. The reason for this is simple: it helps submerge the vegetables that would otherwise float to the top and potentially spoil. For the cover I use a plate as large as I can find. Flea markets and antique shops are great places to find both crocks and plates of different sizes to fit.

Then, you'll need a weight. I sometimes use a bowl filled with water to sit on top of the plate, but you can also use a rock that has been scrubbed and boiled for at least fifteen minutes. A one-gallon glass jug tends to be a great weight for larger crocks, and mason jars filled with water make good weights for smaller crocks or bowls.

. . . .

2 small to medium heads green cabbage, shredded

3 tablespoons unrefined fine sea salt or 6 tablespoons unrefined coarse sea salt (do not use iodized salt, as it can interfere with the culturing process)

1 quart/liter filtered, unchlorinated water

. . . .

In a large, clean crock or large bowl place the green cabbage, pushing down with your clean fist or a wooden spoon to make it more compact and to release the juices as you go. In a pitcher or large measuring cup, dissolve the sea salt in the water, stirring if necessary to encourage the salt to dissolve. Pour over the cabbage in the crock until the ingredients are submerged, leaving a couple of inches at the top for the ingredients to expand.

Place a plate that fits inside the crock over the cabbage-water mixture, and weigh it down with food-safe weights or a bowl or jar of water until the vegetables are submerged under the water-salt brine. Cover with a lid or cloth. Let ferment for at least a week, checking periodically to ensure the cabbage mixture is still submerged below the saltwater brine.

If any mold forms on the surface, simply scoop it out; it will not spoil the sauerkraut. It may form where the mixture meets the air but should not form deeper inside the crock. Of course, if you see mold inside the crock, throw out the contents, thoroughly clean the crock, and start over.

After one week or longer if preferred, dish out the sauerkraut into jars or a bowl and place in the fridge, where it will last for at least a few months.

Apple-Cabbage Kraut

Servings: 20 (approximately 1 cup each)

This is my husband, Curtis's, favorite sauerkraut. He eats it so much that I jokingly started referring to him as Krautis. I love that this sauerkraut not only tastes amazing; it also turns a brilliant pink color that is a gorgeous and bright addition to any plate. Enjoy it on its own or as a delicious condiment on top of salad, hot dogs, sausages, burgers, or over a bowl of brown or black rice. Curtis puts it on most of his sandwiches and wraps or as a side dish for most meals.

1 small to medium head green cabbage, shredded

1 small to medium head purple cabbage, shredded

2 apples of your choice, thinly sliced

2 teaspoons juniper berries, coarsely cracked with a mortar and pestle or pepper mill

3 tablespoons unrefined fine sea salt or 6 tablespoons unrefined coarse sea salt

1 quart/liter filtered, unchlorinated water

In a large, clean crock or large bowl, layer the green cabbage, purple cabbage, apples, and juniper berries until full or until you've used up these ingredients. Using a wooden spoon or your clean fist, punch down the cabbage and apple mixture to make it more compact and to release the juices.

In a pitcher or large measuring cup, dissolve the sea salt in the water, stirring if necessary to encourage the salt to dissolve. Pour over the cabbage-apple mixture in the crock until the ingredients are submerged, leaving a couple of inches at the top for the ingredients to expand.

Place a plate that fits inside the crock over the cabbage-water mixture, and weigh it down with food-safe weights or a bowl or jar of water until the vegetables are submerged under the saltwater brine. Cover with a lid or cloth. Let ferment for at least a week, checking periodically to ensure the cabbage mixture is still submerged below the saltwater brine.

If any mold forms on the surface, simply scoop it out; it will not spoil the sauerkraut. It may form where the mixture meets the air but not deeper inside the crock.

After one week or longer if preferred, dish out the sauerkraut into jars or a bowl and place in the fridge, where it will last for a few months at least.

Cultured Anise Carrots

Servings: 10 (approximately ⅔ cup each)

Just one carrot contains 13,500 IU of beta carotene, which translates into a tremendous amount of nutritional power against free radicals. Beta carotene is anticancerous, prevents cellular damage and premature aging, and is important to prevent cataracts. Combined with digestion-enhancing anise seeds, this is a winning recipe for health that also tastes great. The first time I made and tried Cultured Anise Carrots I was pleasantly surprised how good carrots taste with a slight anise flavor. If you haven't tried anise before, it has a mild licorice-type taste. Serve these carrots on their own as a type of carrot slaw, atop a green salad, within a wrap, or on a sandwich.

1½ pounds carrots, grated

1 teaspoon anise seeds

1 tablespoon sea salt, finely ground, or 2 tablespoons coarsely ground sea salt

3 cups whey, or enough to cover carrot-anise mixture (see Dairy-Free Yogurt recipe on page 186).

In a 1-quart/1-liter wide-mouthed mason jar with a lid, layer the grated carrots, anise seeds, and salt. Add enough whey to cover. Using a small dish, ramekin, or clean weight that fits inside the jar, weigh down the carrots until they are submerged under the liquid. Culture for 3 to 7 days, or longer if you prefer a tangier taste. Lasts about 6 months in the refrigerator.

Green Chili Hot Sauce

Yield: approximately 1 cup

It is simple to make your own probiotic-rich fermented hot sauce. You can use any type of chili you prefer. Jalapeños tend to be a milder chili, Thai red chilies are hotter, and habañeros tend to be superhot. Just choose the chili you prefer depending on the heat level you wish to obtain for your hot sauce. Just a dash or small spoonful is all you will need to add some spice and probiotics to your favorite foods. Be careful when you're working with the chilies to use gloves or wash your hands thoroughly afterward and when opening the food processor or putting the chili puree into a jar; in addition to being a possible skin or eye irritant, it can give off fumes that can irritate the lungs.

5 jalapeño peppers, stems removed

10 Thai red chilies, stems removed

⅓ cup whey (the clearish-yellowish liquid leftover from making yogurt or dairy-free yogurt)

½ teaspoon unrefined sea salt

Puree all ingredients together in a food processor until somewhat smooth. Pour the mixture into a small glass jar with a lid. Cover with the lid, and leave undisturbed for at least 24 hours. Lasts about 6 months in the refrigerator.

Garlic Chili Green Bean Pickles

Servings: 8 to 10 (approximately 10 beans each)

This is a simple recipe that can ensure you always have delicious veggie pickles in the fridge to accompany any meal or to serve as a delicious, healthy, probiotic-rich snack. I created it one summer when I had an unusually large number of beans come up in my garden. Curtis and I couldn't keep up with them, so I came up with the idea of pickling them so we could eat them year-round. The chilies impart a slight spiciness to the beans, while the garlic adds a delicious mild garlic pickle flavor. You can also use the garlic cloves in your favorite dishes or eat them on their own. They will lose some of their intensity to the brine during the fermentation process. I make a large amount and keep them on hand when I'm feeling lazy but want to include a vegetable dish in my meal.

1 to 2 pounds green beans, washed and tops trimmed

3 dried or fresh chilies of your choice (cayenne works well)

3 garlic cloves, cut in half

1 teaspoon coriander seeds

2 to 3 cups filtered, unchlorinated water

2 tablespoons coarse sea salt or 1 tablespoon fine sea salt

Pack green beans, chilies, garlic, and coriander seeds into a 1-quart/1-liter canning jar with a lid, fitting them as tightly as possible. Add water and salt to cover. Cover the jar with a smaller jar or ramekin that fits inside the canning jar as closely as possible to the mouth size; this smaller jar or ramekin will help keep the beans and other ingredients submerged in the brine. Allow to ferment for at least 1 week. Lasts approximately 6 months in the refrigerator.

Fermented Onions

Servings: 10 (approximately 3 tablespoons each)

Fermenting onions mellows their flavor, making them a great addition to wraps, sandwiches, or salads. I love these fermented onions on a Greek-style veggie wrap or on top of hummus and pita wedges. The onion flavor becomes milder during the fermentation process, so don't let the thought of raw onions in this delicious condiment scare you off.

2 small onions, thinly sliced

1 tablespoon fine sea salt or 2 tablespoons coarse sea salt

1 to 2 cups whey, or enough to cover

Layer the onions with the salt in a 1-quart/1-liter wide-mouthed mason jar with a lid. Add enough whey to cover. Seal the jar with the lid, and let ferment for 3 to 7 days. Longer fermentation times mellow the onion flavor and add a naturally tart taste. Lasts approximately 6 months in the refrigerator.

Kimchi (Fermented Cabbage and Vegetable Condiment)

Yield: about 6 cups

Kimchi is a fermented cabbage, vegetable, and spice condiment that is so popular in Korea that it is recognized as the country's national dish. There are countless variations on this condiment, but most tend to have napa cabbage, daikon or radishes, onions or scallions, garlic, ginger, and red peppers or red chilies. Most traditional versions of kimchi include fish sauce, which you can add if you like, but be sure it is free of any preservatives, as they can interfere with the natural fermentation process. This is a vegan version, free of fish sauce. It takes about thirty minutes to prepare and at least a week to ferment, although you can ferment it longer if you prefer.

3 tablespoons unrefined, coarse sea salt or
  1½ tablespoons fine sea salt

3 cups filtered, unchlorinated water

1 pound napa or Chinese cabbage, coarsely chopped

3 heads baby bok choy or 1 large head bok choy
  (approximately 1 pound), coarsely chopped

4 radishes, coarsely chopped

1 small onion

3 cloves garlic

1 2-inch piece ginger

3 chilies

Mix together the water and sea salt until the salt has dissolved to form the brine. Set aside.

Coarsely chop the cabbage, bok choy, and radishes. Mix together, and place in a small crock or bowl. Pour the brine over the vegetable mixture until covered. Place a plate that just fits inside the crock or bowl, and weigh it down with food-grade weights, a jar, or another bowl filled with water. Cover and let sit for at least 4 hours or overnight.

Puree the onion, garlic, ginger, and chilies in a food processor to form a paste.

Drain the brine off the vegetables, reserving it for later use. Taste the vegetable mixture for saltiness. Rinse it if it is too salty-tasting or add a pinch of sea salt if necessary. Mix the vegetables and the spice mixture until thoroughly combined. Pack it tightly into a small crock or bowl, adding a small amount of the brine if necessary to keep the vegetables submerged. Weigh down the vegetables with a plate and a food-grade weight. (I use a smaller glass or ceramic bowl filled with the remaining brine to act as a weight. If you require additional brine or the vegetable mixture expands to reach the bowl, it contains the same brine.) Cover with a lid. Ferment for about 1 week, or longer if you prefer a tangier-tasting kimchi. Place in a glass bowl or jar with a lid and refrigerate. Serve as a side dish, condiment, or atop brown rice over vermicelli noodles for a quick and delicious dinner. Lasts approximately 6 months in the refrigerator.

Desserts

Cultured Coconut Cream

Yield: approximately 1 cup

Cultured coconut cream is a delicious, rich, and probiotic-rich cream that is the perfect replacement for dairy whipped cream. It contains all the benefits of coconut milk, including its medium chain triglycerides (MCTs) that have been found to be helpful for weight loss, thyroid imbalances, and other health issues. Top pancakes, waffles, fruit salad, or other dishes with this delicious creamy treat. Alternatively, use it as a sweet dip for fruit slices or atop a bowl of fresh berries.

> **1 13.5-ounce can coconut milk (regular, not the "light" or low-fat version), shaken well**
>
> **1 capsule or ¼ teaspoon probiotic powder**

Pour the coconut milk into a small glass bowl. (Do not use metal bowls, as they can inhibit the culturing process.) Cover with a clean cloth, and leave in an undisturbed, warm setting for 8 to 10 hours. Cover with a lid and refrigerate.

After the coconut cream has cooled for at least an hour or two, it is ready for use. Use only the upper portion of cream, as it has thickened. The lower coconut water/milk portion can be saved and added to smoothies, juices, or as a "starter" to culture other foods. Lasts approximately 1 week in the refrigerator.

Vanilla Coconut Cream

Yield: approximately 1 cup

This rich and delicious cream is an excellent alternative to the dairy versions. It has a sweet vanilla-coconut flavor and is great served wherever you'd normally use whipped cream, including over fruit, on pancakes or waffles, or atop your favorite dessert.

Notes on ingredients: Vanilla powder is not the same as vanilla sugar. Vanilla powder is ground vanilla beans and is available in most health food stores or by grinding your own from fresh vanilla beans.

1 batch of Cultured Coconut Cream (page 216)

1 to 2 teaspoons honey or pure maple syrup

1 teaspoon vanilla powder or pure vanilla extract

Drain the clearish liquid—whey—off the Cultured Coconut Cream; reserve whey as a "starter" for other recipes. Use only the thick coconut cream.

Add the honey and vanilla powder. Stir together until combined. Serve. It keeps for a week or two in a glass or ceramic bowl, covered with a lid, in the refrigerator.

Dairy-Free Cream

Yield: approximately 1½ cups

This cream is delicious served over fresh fruit or on top of pancakes or waffles. It is rich in calcium, magnesium, and probiotics and is a healthier alternative to the dairy version.

1 cup almond milk

½ cup raw, unsalted cashews

> **2 fresh Medjool dates, pitted**
>
> **1 capsule probiotic powder**

. . . .

Blend the almond milk, cashews, and dates together until smooth. Open the end of the probiotic capsule, and add the contents to the almond milk–cashew mixture; stir until mixed. Pour into a glass or ceramic bowl, and cover with a lid or clean cloth. Leave in a warm location for at least 2 hours. Stir before serving. Lasts approximately 1 week in the refrigerator.

Vanilla Coconut Ice Cream

. . . .

Servings: 4 (approximately 1 cup or 1 pop each)

This delicious, nutritious, and naturally low-sugar ice cream is the perfect treat for a hot day. The almond milk packs plenty of calcium and magnesium, while the coconut milk is rich in medium chain triglycerides (MCTs) that boost metabolism and help reset the thyroid gland. This version is also rich in natural probiotic cultures to give your GI tract and total body a boost. To keep the ice cream healthier and low in sugar, I use only two fresh dates, but you can add more if you prefer a sweeter-tasting ice cream.

Note on ingredients: Vanilla powder is not the same as vanilla sugar. Vanilla powder is ground vanilla beans and is available in most health food stores or by grinding your own from fresh vanilla beans.

. . . .

> **1 13.5-ounce can coconut milk (not the "light" version), shaken well**
>
> **1 probiotic capsule or ¼ teaspoon probiotic powder**
>
> **2½ cups almond milk**
>
> **2 fresh Medjool dates, pitted, more if you desire a sweeter ice cream**
>
> **1 teaspoon vanilla powder or pure vanilla extract**

. . . .

Empty the coconut milk into a small bowl with a lid. Add the contents of the probiotic capsule by removing one end or add the probiotic powder; stir together. Cover and allow to ferment for at least 1 to 2 hours, but preferably longer; 8 to 10 hours or overnight is ideal.

Blend together all the ingredients, including the cultured coconut milk and liquid whey (if it has separated). Pour into an ice cream maker, and make according to manufacturer's directions, usually 25 to 30 minutes in the machine. Alternatively, pour into a popsicle mold and add sticks. Let freeze for a few hours or until frozen. Run hot water over the mold until pops loosen. Serve immediately or store in the freezer for up to 1 week.

Creamsicle Ice Cream

Servings: 4 (approximately 1 cup or 1 pop each)

This light orange–colored ice cream is as delicious as it is beautiful. It tastes like the creamsicles I ate as a child but is so much healthier. It is high in vitamin C, protein, calcium, magnesium, and, of course, health-boosting probiotics. If you don't have an ice cream machine, pour into pop molds for delicious creamsicles.

¾ cup raw, unsalted cashews

1 cup filtered, unchlorinated water

1 probiotic capsule or ½ teaspoon probiotic powder

5 mandarin oranges, peeled, seeded

1 cup almond milk

2 fresh Medjool dates, pitted

1 teaspoon vanilla powder or pure vanilla extract

Blend together the cashews and water; pour into a small glass or ceramic bowl. Add the contents of the probiotic capsule or the probiotic powder, then cover and let ferment for 8 to 12 hours.

Blend together the fermented cashew mixture, mandarin oranges, almond milk, dates, and vanilla until creamy. Pour into an ice cream maker, and make according to manufacturer's directions, usually 25 to 30 minutes in the machine. Alternatively, pour into a popsicle mold and add sticks. Let freeze for a few hours or until frozen. Run hot water over the mold until pops loosen. Serve immediately or store in freezer for up to 1 week.

Black and Blue Berry Gelato

Servings: 4 (approximately 1 cup or 1 pop each)

This gelato not only tastes amazing; it is a nutritional powerhouse. Packed with vitamin C, blackberries also contain ellagic acid, an important phytonutrient that protects skin cells from damaging UV rays. Ellagic acid prevents the breakdown of collagen in the skin that naturally occurs as we age and is linked to wrinkling. Many phytonutrients give blueberries their dark blue color, rich flavor, and disease-fighting phytonutrients, including anthocyanins, ellagic acid, quercetin, and catechins. Blueberries are showing tremendous promise in preventing and treating brain disease thanks to their proven ability to reduce heat shock proteins that are linked with Alzheimer's and Parkinson's disease as well as other neurological disorders. The lemon zest contains limonene, one of nature's most potent anticancer compounds—this is a superb anticancer treat. If you don't have an ice cream machine, pour into pop molds for fruit-flavored pops.

½ cup raw, unsalted cashews

1 cup blackberries, fresh or frozen

1 cup blueberries

½ lemon, juiced and zested

1¼ cups almond milk

2 apples, cored

1 tablespoon honey, D-ribose, or other sweetener

Blend all ingredients together in a blender. Pour into an ice cream maker, and make according to manufacturer's directions, usually 25 to 30 minutes in the machine. Alternatively, pour into a popsicle mold and add sticks. Let freeze for a few hours or until frozen. Run hot water over the mold until pops loosen. Serve or store in freezer for up to 1 week.

Vanilla Frozen Yogurt

Servings: 3 (approximately 1 cup each)

This simple and delicious frozen yogurt is packed with probiotics, as most of the commercial varieties don't contain live cultures. The amount of dates is for a low-sugar frozen yogurt; if you prefer a sweeter frozen yogurt, simply increase the number of dates used.

Note on ingredients: Vanilla powder is not the same as vanilla sugar. Vanilla powder is ground vanilla beans and is available in most health food stores or by grinding your own from fresh vanilla beans.

2½ cups almond milk, unsweetened

½ cup raw, unsalted cashews

2 fresh Medjool dates, pitted

1 capsule probiotics or ½ teaspoon probiotic powder

1 teaspoon vanilla powder or pure vanilla extract

Blend together the almond milk, cashews, and dates until smooth and creamy. Pour into a medium-large glass or ceramic bowl. Empty the contents of the probiotic capsule or probiotic powder into the mixture and stir until mixed. Cover and let rest in a warm, undisturbed location for at least 2 hours but preferably longer. Pour the mixture into an ice cream maker, and make according to manufacturer's directions until it reaches the desired consistency. Serve or store in freezer for up to 1 week.

Mango Frozen Yogurt Pops

Servings: 4 pops

These frozen yogurt pops are cooling on a hot day. Plus, they are packed with probiotics from the dairy-free yogurt and are naturally sweet, thanks to the mango. You can use either dairy-based yogurt or one of the dairy-free yogurts above—the Sweet Yogurt recipe works well.

1 cup of yogurt of your choice

1 mango (alternatively, use 1 cup of frozen mango), peeled, pitted, and chopped

1 teaspoon honey or agave, optional

Blend all ingredients together until smooth. Pour into a mold. Freeze. Run hot water over the mold until pops loosen. Serve or store in freezer for up to 1 week.

Coconut Ice Cream

Servings: 4 (approximately 1 cup or 1 pop each)

This ice cream is perfect on a hot summer's day, but it is so good that you'll want to enjoy it year-round. It is packed with probiotics found in the Cultured Coconut Milk. The cashews add protein, and the dates add natural sweetness along with fiber and minerals. If you don't have an ice cream machine, simply pour into a pop mold to make delicious probiotic-rich coconut pops.

Note on ingredients: Vanilla powder is not the same as vanilla sugar. Vanilla powder is ground vanilla beans and is available in most health food stores or by grinding your own from fresh vanilla beans.

. . . .

1 batch Cultured Coconut Milk (page 195)

½ cup raw, unsalted cashews

2 to 3 fresh Medjool dates, pitted (or use more, depending on the level of sweetness you prefer)

2 teaspoons vanilla powder or extract

. . . .

Blend all ingredients together until smooth. Pour into an ice cream maker, and make according to manufacturer's directions. Serve immediately when frozen. Alternatively, pour into a popsicle mold and add sticks. Let freeze for a few hours or until frozen. Run hot water over the mold until pops loosen. Serve or store in freezer for up to 1 week.

Metric Conversions

The recipes in this book have not been tested with metric measurements, so some variations might occur.

Remember that the weight of dry ingredients varies according to the volume or density factor: 1 cup of flour weighs far less than 1 cup of sugar, and 1 tablespoon doesn't necessarily hold 3 teaspoons.

General Formula for Metric Conversion

Ounces to grams	multiply ounces by 28.35
Grams to ounces	multiply ounces by 0.035
Pounds to grams	multiply pounds by 453.5
Pounds to kilograms	multiply pounds by 0.45
Cups to liters	multiply cups by 0.24
Fahrenheit to Celsius	subtract 32 from Fahrenheit temperature, multiply by 5, divide by 9
Celsius to Fahrenheit	multiply Celsius temperature by 9, divide by 5, add 32

Volume (Liquid) Measurements

1 teaspoon = ⅙ fluid ounce = 5 milliliters

1 tablespoon = ½ fluid ounce = 15 milliliters

2 tablespoons = 1 fluid ounce = 30 milliliters

¼ cup = 2 fluid ounces = 60 milliliters

⅓ cup = 2⅔ fluid ounces = 79 milliliters

½ cup = 4 fluid ounces = 118 milliliters

1 cup or ½ pint = 8 fluid ounces = 250 milliliters

2 cups or 1 pint = 16 fluid ounces = 500 milliliters

4 cups or 1 quart = 32 fluid ounces = 1,000 milliliters

1 gallon = 4 liters

Volume (Dry) Measurements

¼ teaspoon = 1 milliliter

½ teaspoon = 2 milliliters

¾ teaspoon = 4 milliliters

1 teaspoon = 5 milliliters

1 tablespoon = 15 milliliters

¼ cup = 59 milliliters

⅓ cup = 79 milliliters

½ cup = 118 milliliters

⅔ cup = 158 milliliters

¾ cup = 177 milliliters

1 cup = 225 milliliters

4 cups or 1 quart = 1 liter

½ gallon = 2 liters

1 gallon = 4 liters

Weight (Mass) Measurements

1 ounce = 30 grams

2 ounces = 55 grams

3 ounces = 85 grams

4 ounces = ¼ pound = 125 grams

8 ounces = ½ pound = 240 grams

12 ounces = ¾ pound = 375 grams

16 ounces = 1 pound = 454 grams

Linear Measurements

½ in = 1½ cm

1 inch = 2½ cm

6 inches = 15 cm

8 inches = 20 cm

10 inches = 25 cm

12 inches = 30 cm

20 inches = 50 cm

Oven Temperature Equivalents, Fahrenheit (F) and Celsius (C)

100°F = 38°C

200°F = 95°C

250°F = 120°C

300°F = 150°C

350°F = 180°C

400°F = 205°C

450°F = 230°C

Appendix: The Cutting-Edge Research

When the Medicine Is Worse Than the Illness

In Chapter 3 we discussed when medicine is worse than the illness. Additional research shows the following:

Scientists at the Southern California Evidence-Based Practice Center, RAND Health in Santa Monica, California, published a study in the *Journal of the American Medical Association* in which they assessed the research to date on probiotics in treating antibiotic-related diarrhea. They found that the pooled evidence suggests that probiotics are linked to a reduction in antibiotic-associated diarrhea. The probiotic strains reviewed included many *Lactobacillus, Bifidobacterium, Saccharomyces, Streptococcus, Enterococcus,* and/or *Bacillus* bacteria.[1]

In another study published in the *World Journal of Gastroenterology*, researchers found that probiotics were found to be "useful in preventing the adverse effects of antibiotics, modulating the immune response, gastro-protection, and the general promotion of health."[2] So we know that the practice of taking probiotics alongside antibiotics is a good one and supported by research. Probiotics are demonstrating that they can strengthen our immune systems and gastrointestinal tract to reduce the incidence and severity of drug reactions. And other research also supports this conclusion. A study at Gothenburg University in Sweden found that the probiotic *Lactobacillus plantarum*, taken along with antibiotics, reduced the incidence of antibiotic-associated diarrhea, suggesting that this particular strain of probiotic taken during and after antibiotic treatment can help reduce or altogether prevent the negative symptoms of the drugs.[3]

How Probiotics Work

Additionally, *H. pylori* has been shown in studies to affect gene expression in cells of the GI tract to cause reduced mucus secretion. Conversely, research shows that *Lactobacilli plantarum* and *rhamnosus* improve the expression of the genes involved, further inhibiting the ability of harmful bacteria like *H. pylori* to survive.

Healing Ulcers and Gastritis

Here is some additional detail on a study at the Laboratory of Microbiology and Probiotics, Institute of Nutrition and Food Technology, University of Chile, in Santiago, Chile, to assess the possible effects of combining cranberry juice with probiotics to treat *H. pylori* infections:

The researchers divided children infected with *H. pylori* bacteria into four groups: the first group received placebo treatment, the second group received a placebo juice with the probiotic supplement, the third group received cranberry juice with probiotics that had been destroyed by heat, and the fourth group received cranberry juice and live cultures of *L. johnsonii La1* in supplement form. The results were interesting. The placebo group experienced a 1.5 percent rate of *H. pylori* infection elimination; the placebo juice/real probiotic group had a 14.9 percent eradication of infection; the cranberry juice and heat-destroyed probiotic group had a 16.9 percent eradication of *H. pylori*; and the group that was treated with the real cranberry juice and live cultures of probiotics had an eradication rate of 22.9 percent.

More Antibacterial Power of Probiotics

Probiotics may help to prevent skin infections. According to a study by the Dermatology Division of the Department of Medicine at the University of California San Diego in LaJolla, California, the inappropriate use of antibiotics may eliminate the beneficial bacteria that protect the skin, making it more difficult to fight MRSA skin infections.[4]

Groundbreaking Research on a Devastating Disease

Here is some additional detail on the pilot study presented in the journal *Mycopathologia* in which researchers assessed the effects of probiotic supplementation through ingestion of yogurt as a way to affect the Candida infection:

Twenty-four women underwent a sixty-day initiation period, during which they did not consume probiotics, followed by two fifteen-day probiotic consumption periods, each with a thirty-day "washout" phase in between in which they didn't consume probiotics. Mouth and vaginal swabs were collected on days zero, sixty, and seventy-four to assess whether the probiotics had any effect on the Candida infections.

The Inflammation Connection

Here's more information about cytokines and how they are linked with inflammation in the body: Cytokines are cell-signaling, hormone-like molecules that encourage cellular communication in immune responses as well as stimulate the movement of cells toward sites of inflammation, infection, and trauma. Cytokines may affect the cell from which it originated or nearby cells, or it may produce effects throughout the whole body, such as with fevers.[5]

In an effort to better understand the effects of cytokines, researchers conducted a study on healthy adults in which they induced the release of cytokines. They discovered that cytokines, when induced in healthy adults, cause anxiety, symptoms of depression, and cognitive disturbances. They also lower an important compound, brain-derived neurotrophic factor (BDNF), which protects our nerve cells.[6]

Allergies and Allergy-Related Conditions

Probiotics may help regulate the immune system to ward off allergies. Because the mucous membranes are the passageways by which environmental allergens gain access to the body, protecting the mucous membranes by increasing an immune substance known as immunoglobulin A (IgA) helps to create a protective coating against the allergens.[7]

Anxiety and Depression

How inflammation is connected to anxiety and depression: Additional studies show that probiotic bacteria lower negative immune system compounds called "cytokines" (which you may recall from our inflammation discussion) not only in the gut but also throughout the bloodstream. Cytokines are linked to both anxiety and symptoms of depression, among other symptoms in healthy adults.

Arthritis

There is a surprising link between harmful joint infections and arthritis. The researchers analyzed 144 stool samples from rheumatoid arthritis sufferers and healthy controls. They assessed gut bacteria between the two groups using DNA analysis and found that *P. copri* was more abundant in newly diagnosed rheumatoid arthritis patients than it was in healthy individuals or those with an established RA condition.

The NYU researchers built on the understanding established by earlier research published in the *Journal of Clinical Investigation*. In this study mice that were raised in germ-free conditions developed joint inflammation after the introduction of specific harmful gut bacteria. The study author, Dan Littman, MD, PhD, professor of pathology and immunology, said that "studies of rodent models have clearly shown that the intestinal microbiota contribute significantly to the causation of systemic autoimmune diseases."[8]

In a specific form of arthritis known as spondyloarthritis (SpA), the connection between intestinal inflammation and the disease has been extensively studied. Researchers have identified subclinical gut inflammation to be strongly associated with joint inflammation in this condition. Although the research has not yet explored possible probiotic treatments of SpA, the connection remains. Therefore, it may be beneficial to address the gut inflammation with probiotics as part of an overall SpA treatment strategy.

Brain Disease

Probiotics may also help reduce inflammation linked to brain disease. They observed the effects of particular inflammatory compounds called IL-6, which has been found to be elevated in brain disease, suggesting that the probiotics may be helpful in treating brain diseases.[9]

It's All in the Strains—Heart Disease

Here's more information about the ways probiotics may be helpful in treating heart disease. Another probiotic strain is proving itself helpful in reducing high cholesterol levels. Researchers at the Clinic of Geriatric Medicine, Faculty of Medicine at Comenius University in Slovakia, studied the effects of the probiotic strain *Enterococcus faecium* M-74 on cholesterol levels over the course of fifty-six weeks. They administered the probiotic supplement containing 2 billion CFUs once daily. The participants, averaging seventy-four years old, experienced a 20 percent drop in LDL cholesterol and a 12 percent drop in total cholesterol by the end of the study.[10]

Canadian researchers tested still another strain to determine its effectiveness against cholesterol levels and inflammation. The Canadian study published in the *European Journal of Clinical Nutrition* explored the effects of *Lactobacillus reuteri NCIMB 30242* on cholesterol levels and C-reactive protein. The scientists at the Faculty of Medicine at McGill University, in Montreal, Quebec, Canada, found that during the nine-week period of the study cholesterol levels remained the same, but C-reactive protein dropped.[11]

Infant Nutrition

Early administration of certain probiotics may help newborns. Additional research in the *American Journal of Clinical Nutrition* found that infancy is a critical period for the early colonization of beneficial microbes in the almost-sterile gut of newborn infants. The researchers indicated that doing so may provide a good opportunity to prevent later health problems such as allergies and diabetes.[12]

Aging

Probiotics may be helpful to slow or manage conditions linked to aging. A new animal study on male, aging mice may indicate potential for probiotics for aging human men as well. Scientists at the Massachusetts Institute of Technology in various locations in the United States and Greece jointly conducted a study to determine whether adding the probiotic *Lactobacillus reuteri* to the animals' drinking water would have any effect on their levels of the hormone testosterone and preventing shrinking testicular size in aging mice. They found that the mice that routinely consumed the probiotics maintained larger testicles and had higher levels of testosterone in their blood than similarly aged mice that were not fed the probiotics. The scientists concluded that these findings were not only novel but also hold great potential for probiotic therapy to maintain the hormonal and gonadal health typical of much younger healthy individuals, particularly because the use of probiotics has other beneficial health effects compared to drug therapies, which tend to have damaging side effects.[13]

The Straight Goods on Yogurt

Because some yogurts contain the probiotic species *L. delbrueckii bulgaricus*, which is believed to have originated on the surface of a plant, it is believed that milk may have become inadvertently inoculated with a plant containing this bacteria, resulting in fermented milk, or yogurt.[14]

You may find it interesting to note that although we think of yogurt as being solely from cow's milk, many other cultures make yogurt from various types of animal milk, including sheep's, goat's, and camel's milk. Scientists at the University of West Hungary compared yogurt made with these animal milks to assess whether probiotic cultures survived better in certain types of milk. All four products had high levels of *S. thermophilus* probiotics both at the beginning of the study and after forty-two days. The camel's milk, in particular, showed no significant decline in this probiotic, whereas the other yogurts did. Some of the probiotics decreased faster than others. For example, their research showed a slow and constant decrease in *Lactobacilli* probiotic cultures over time in all of the animal milks, including the cow's milk yogurt. All four yogurt types had about the same amount of *Lactobacilli* left after forty-two days in the study, so none of the yogurt was superior in that regard.[15] Should you switch to camel's milk yogurt? Well, that's entirely up to you—if you can even find it. Unfortunately, no comparisons were made between the animal milk yogurt and dairy-free alternatives.

The Problems with Most Dairy Products

Research links the consumption of dairy products with the formation of arthritis. In one study of rabbits, scientist Richard Panush was able to produce inflamed joints in the animals by switching their water to cow's milk. In another study scientists observed more than a 50 percent reduction in the pain and swelling of arthritis when participants eliminated milk and dairy products from their diet.

Alternatives to Dairy Yogurt

The College of Human Ecology at Yonsei University in Seoul, South Korea, conducted an interesting study exploring the effects of a high-cholesterol diet on rats. They divided the rats into groups in which one group ate 20 percent casein, a milk protein, while the other two groups ate soy milk or fermented soy milk to comprise 20 percent of the total diet. Then the researchers examined the rats to determine any health differences. They found that the soy groups both had lower liver cholesterol levels and blood triglycerides than the dairy group. High cholesterol and blood triglycerides are indicators of heart disease, so reducing them can improve heart health. Only the rats that ate the fermented soy had reduced liver triglyceride levels, increased blood HDL cholesterol levels (the "good" cholesterol), and higher amounts of fecal cholesterol, an indicator that their bodies were eliminating more harmful cholesterol in their stools. The researchers concluded that including fermented soy in the diet may be a way to enhance the beneficial effect of soy on fat metabolism.[16] And considering their results, this study also suggests that soy yogurt consumption may be a great way to improve heart health.

A study at the Department of Food Science and Nutrition, Mukogawa Women's University, in Hyogo, Japan, found that rats fed a high-cholesterol diet and probiotic-fermented soy yogurt had improved liver weight and fat mass than the rats that only ate the high-cholesterol diet. The yogurt-eating group also had a significant reduction in cholesterol levels compared to the control group. The researchers concluded that fermented soy milk can regulate cholesterol metabolism in animals fed a high-cholesterol diet.[17]

Another study conducted at the Institute of Food Science, Technology and Nutrition (ICTAN-CSIC), in Madrid, Spain, found that several bacteria from the *Enterococcus* family increased the availability of isoflavones during the fermentation of soy yogurt. They found that the probiotics also increased the antioxidant and anti-inflammatory potential of soy milk and concluded that regularly eating soy yogurt "could be a promising strategy in the prevention therapy against cardiovascular disease."[18]

The Great Soy Debate

The study I mentioned earlier from the *International Journal of Food Sciences and Nutrition* found that dairy yogurt increased the absorption of isoflavones from soy milk. Unfortunately, the scientists didn't assess the effects of eating yogurt made from soy milk, as I believe the beneficial results would have been similar or superior for soy yogurt. After all, isoflavones are *found* in soy milk, not dairy milk, and the culturing process is known to improve absorbability of nutrients, as the Yonsei University researchers proved.

Soy Yogurt and Osteoporosis

Scientists at the National Taiwan University in Taipei, Taiwan, published a study exploring soy yogurt's effects on bone mineral density, which they published in the *Journal of Agricultural Food Chemistry*. The soy milk was fermented with *Lactobacillus paracasei* and *plantarum*. One group of female animals without ovaries were fed the resulting soy yogurt for eight weeks, while the other group ate their standard diet without the addition of soy yogurt. They found that the mice that ate the soy yogurt had a significant increase in bone density and thickness over the mice that didn't eat the soy yogurt. The researchers also found that the *Lactobacilli* increased the isoflavone, soluble calcium, and vitamin D_3 content of the soy milk. The researchers concluded that the soy yogurt may reduce bone loss and lower the risk of osteoporosis in animals.[19] The same scientists conducted a follow-up study to retest their results over six weeks using the same probiotics to create soy yogurt. Again, they found that the bones were significantly denser in the soy yogurt group of animals than the control group. They also found that there was less breakdown of bone in the soy yogurt group than the control group, a process known as resorption.

Kefir—Vitamin Boost

Over one hundred years ago the Nobel Prize–winning Russian biologist, zoologist, and protozoologist Elie Metchnikoff found that kefir activates the flow of saliva and stimulates peristalsis and digestive juices in the intestinal tract, all of which could account for its digestion-improving abilities.[20] Peristalsis is the process of contraction and relaxation of the muscles in the walls of the digestive tract to propel digested food forward and aid elimination of waste.

Other Conditions

One probiotic, *Lactobacillus kefiranofaciens*, has been found to produce a substance known as kefiran.[21] In a study conducted at the Research and Development Division, Daiwa Pharmaceutical Company, in Tokyo, Japan, and published in the journal *Biofactors*, researchers found that kefiran from kefir prevented increases in blood pressure, reduced cholesterol levels, and lowered blood glucose levels in animals.

In a study presented in the *International Journal of Obesity*, researchers at Da-Yeh and National Chung Hsing Universities assessed the effects of kefir consumption on fatty liver disease. Fatty liver disease is a common problem linked with being overweight and obesity, insulin resistance, and diabetes. Unfortunately, there is no medical treatment that is effective for this health problem, so the researchers attempted to find new and natural strategies to improve the condition. They found that daily kefir consumption improved fatty liver syndrome and specific metabolic issues linked to the disease, including increased metabolic rate, improved energy expenditure, and decreased triglyceride and cholesterol in the liver. The scientists concluded that kefir could potentially prevent or treat fatty liver disease.[22]

A fatty liver is surprisingly common and is a hidden factor in weight that just won't budge. Here are some of the signs you might have a fatty liver: being overweight, particularly in the abdomen; difficulty losing weight; type 2 diabetes; exhaustion; immune system problems; elevated triglycerides or cholesterol in your blood; and a diagnosis of Syndrome X or metabolic syndrome.

Magic Miso—Cancer

Scientists assessed miso consumption on spontaneous or radiation-induced liver tumors in animals fed miso for thirteen months. Their research, published in the *International Journal of Oncology*, showed that the miso significantly reduced the frequency and number of liver tumors in the male animals but, surprisingly, not the females. The scientists were not certain why miso protected the males but not the females but believe hormonal factors may be involved. More research is needed to understand their findings, but in the meantime their results could have promise for preventing and possibly reversing liver tumors in men.[23]

In a study published in the *Journal of the National Cancer Institute*, researchers found that regular miso consumption could reduce the risk of breast cancer in women by up to 54 percent.[24] The reduced risk was especially high in postmenopausal women. Research in the *Japanese Journal of Cancer Research* also demonstrated miso's protective effect against breast cancer.[25] Additional research at the Department of Cancer Research at Hiroshima University found that miso consumption at the beginning of cancer treatment could even reduce the occurrence of breast tumors as effectively as the cancer drug tamoxifen.[26] That's great news for anyone suffering from cancer. Of course, you should work with your physician when making important medical decisions, such as those involving cancer treatment.

In another study at Hiroshima University in Hiroshima, Japan, researchers tested miso fermented for 4 days, 120 days, or 180 days to determine its effects against radiation. They found the best results were obtained with 180-day fermented miso, which inhibited colon, lung, breast, and liver tumors in mice exposed to radiation, suggesting that miso may protect against radiation injury and that the longer fermentation time may increase the anticancer effects of miso consumption.[27] The researchers found that when miso was fed to mice after the radiation exposures, the miso didn't have the same effects. They concluded that to reap miso's radiation protection benefits, the blood must contain a certain concentration of the active compounds in miso prior to radiation exposure.[28]

What Happens During Sauerkraut and Other Vegetable Fermentation?

A study at MTT Agrifood Research, Finland, and published in the *Journal of Agricultural and Food Chemistry* found that the fermentation process breaks down compounds known as glucosinolates found in cabbage into a more bio-active form of the nutrients called isothiocyanates, which are known to fight cancer.[29] According to one of the authors, Eeva-Liisa Ryhanen, "We are finding that fermented cabbage could be healthier than raw or cooked cabbage, especially for fighting cancer."[30]

According to Leonard Bjeldanes, professor of food toxicology at the University of California at Berkeley, "The cancer rates come down as much as 40 percent when you go from low consumption of (sauerkraut) to high consumption."[31] Although he didn't specify how much constitutes low or high consumption, considering that North Americans eat virtually no sauerkraut in which the cultures are alive, moderate daily consumption may be sufficient to attain this cancer reduction.

Pass the Kimchi

The scientists isolated *Lactobacillus plantarum* (strain *DK119*, specifically), crediting the beneficial bacteria for its antiviral action. The researchers found that animals treated with the probiotic had lowered viral loads in the lungs and reduced inflammation. They also found that the amount ingested made a difference. Those animals given the highest amounts of the *Lactobacillus plantarum* bacteria had the best immunity against the flu virus when scientists exposed them to it.

Additionally, scientists at the Department of Life and Nanopharmaceutical Sciences, Kyung Hee University, in Seoul, South Korea, found a probiotic strain unique to kimchi during their microbiological assessments of the many probiotics contained in kimchi. After further assessing the "new" probiotic's genetic composition, they named it *Lactobacillus pentosus var. plantarum C29* because it closely resembled both *L. pentosus* and *L. plantarum.*

Dermatitis simply means skin inflammation or irritation. It is a common problem, but this new research published in the *Journal of Applied Microbiology* shows promise for treating the condition from the source of the inflammation rather than just the symptoms by applying creams or ointments.[32]

Researchers at the Department of Food and Nutrition and Institute of Health Sciences, Korea University, South Korea, varied the amount of salt used in making kimchi from 1.4 percent to 3.0 percent of the wet weight of ingredients. There was no increase in blood pressure in the hypertensive rats that ate the low-sodium kimchi (1.4 percent of the wet weight of the other ingredients).[33] The lower amount of sodium is still sufficient to keep harmful microorganisms at bay while encouraging the proliferation of beneficial probiotics, particularly in an environment deprived of oxygen.

Kombucha for Wound Treatment

Kombucha also demonstrated effectiveness at treating wounds in animal studies. Researchers at the Department of Pathology, Faculty of Veterinary Medicine, Tehran University, in Iran, found that kombucha was slightly more effective than a medical ointment typically used for skin infections linked to burns or wounds. In the study the researchers divided the animals into two groups: in one group nitrofurazone ointment was applied, and in the other group, kombucha. The researchers assessed the healing of wounds and found that kombucha encouraged healing slightly more than the ointment did. They also observed more inflammation in the nitrofurazone group than in the kombucha group.[34]

Perhaps one of the most unusual studies exploring the possible uses of kombucha involved spraying it into the lungs of animals that had been exposed to silica dust. The purpose of the study was to explore possible therapy options for miners who are exposed to silica dust on a regular basis. The animals were then given treatment with either a drug used for this purpose or by inhaling two different types of kombucha. The free silica levels in the lungs of animals treated with kombucha were significantly lower than those for any other silica-exposed group. These preliminary results indicate that inhaling kombucha preparations promoted the discharge of silica dust from lung tissues. Although more research is definitely needed, researchers concluded that kombucha inhalation may be a useful new treatment for lung diseases that result from breathing in silica dust and other lung diseases resulting from breathing in dust from coal, graphite, or man-made carbon, particularly from mining.[35]

In a study conducted at the College of Engineering, China Agricultural University, Beijing, China, and published in the *Journal of the Science of Food and Agriculture*, researchers explored the liver-protective properties of kombucha to determine which microorganism(s) and chemical constituents might be responsible for these protective effects. In this study researchers assessed kombucha's ability to protect the animals against liver injury resulting from acetaminophen (Tylenol is one of the main brand names of acetaminophen). They attributed the liver-protecting effects to a chemical compound made by *Gluconacetobacter sp. A4* bacteria found in kombucha tea.[36]

There are both bacteria and yeasts involved in the fermentation of the sweetened tea into kombucha, including *Gluconacetobacter*, which laboratory analysis found to be the dominant bacteria present in kombucha tea (sometimes greater than 85 percent of the bacteria), *Lactobacilli* (up to 30 percent of the bacteria), and trace amounts of *Acetobacter* (less than 2 percent). The yeast populations are dominated by *Zygosaccharomyces*, which comprises more than 95 percent of yeast in the fermented beverage.[37]

Resources

More Information About Dr. Michelle Schoffro Cook

World's Healthiest News
Subscribe to Dr. Schoffro Cook's free e-zine, *World's Healthiest News*, to get the latest natural health insights, news, research, recipes, and more. Each edition features concise information you can immediately use to boost your energy, enhance detoxification, supercharge your immune system, and look and feel great. You'll find delicious and nutritious recipes as well as cutting-edge research on nutrition, disease prevention, and healing. You'll also get exclusive deals on some of your favorite health products and discover health tips that you can apply to your life today—all from a source you can trust and at a price you can't beat: FREE! Subscribe at www.WorldsHealthiestDiet.com.

Dr. Michelle's Blogs
Follow Dr. Michelle's popular blogs at:
    www.DrMichelleCook.com
    www.HealthySurvivalist.com
    www.PureFoodWarrior.com
    www.care2.com/greenliving/author/mcook

Where to Find Cultures and Supplies

Most health food stores carry a range of cultured foods, starter cultures, and supplies you will need to begin. If you can't find them locally, there are some excellent online suppliers.

Upaya Naturals

www.upayanaturals.com

It can be difficult to find water kefir grains, but Upaya Naturals offers dehydrated grains to help you get started making nondairy and juice kefir.

GEM Cultures

www.gemcultures.com

Gem Cultures sells kefir grains, kombucha mothers, and many other cultures to help you get started.

South River Miso Company

www.southrivermiso.com

The South River Miso Company offers starter kits for making miso.

Sprout Master

www.sproutmaster.com

Sprout Master offers kombucha mothers and kombucha-making equipment within Canada.

The Tempeh Lab

www.thefarmcommunity.com/business-Tempeh_Lab.html

If you're interested in making tempeh, the Tempeh Lab has everything you need to get started.

Kombucha Kamp

www.kombuchakamp.com

Kombucha Kamp offers live kombucha cultures and full kits with everything you need to get started making kombucha.

Real Raw Foods

www.rawrealfood.com

Real Raw Foods offers raw, organic cashews and almonds for many of the recipes contained in this book.

Equipment

The Probiotic Jar

www.TheProbioticJar.com

The Probiotic Jar makes fermenting your own foods simple, almost foolproof, and ensures that you always have probiotic-rich foods readily available.

VitaClay

vitaclaychef.com

The VitaClay is an electric yogurt maker, rice cooker, and slow cooker all in one device. Unlike devices that use metal containers coated in an unhealthy coating, this one uses a clay pot, making it a healthier alternative. For more information check out my websites www.DrMichelleCook.com and www.TheProbioticPromise.com.

Genetically Modified Foods

For more information about genetically modified foods, follow Dr. Cook's blogs and check out her book *Weekend Wonder Detox* and the website www.seeds ofdeception.com.

The Environmental Working Group is a Washington, DC–based environmental organization that specializes in research and advocacy in the areas of toxic chemicals, agricultural subsidies, public lands, and corporate accountability. See their website at www.ewg.org.

Water Filtration

Most cultured foods require purified water. Chlorine that is routinely used in municipal water treatment kills beneficial bacteria and will stunt their growth, causing many of the recipes to fail. If you don't have the budget for an extensive water filtration unit, there are many excellent and affordable options.

There are many different types of water filtration systems, including activated carbon (like Brita), reverse osmosis, ultraviolet (UV) systems, distillation, water ionizers, and water alkalinizers. They vary greatly in the toxins they remove from water. To help you navigate the different types of water filtration system available, here is a brief overview.

Activated carbon can absorb thousands of different toxic compounds. They are available in under-the counter models, pitchers, and water bottles.

Reverse osmosis is highly effective against bacteria, viruses, arsenic, fluoride, nitrates, and most of the substances captured by activated carbon.

Ultraviolet (UV) light is a form of radiation that kills viruses, mold, algae, bacteria, and yeasts; however, it doesn't work well against heavy metals. As a result it is often combined with other forms of filtration.

Distillation removes all minerals, including beneficial ones, from water. Although many health practitioners love distilled water, I'm not a fan. I feel it is essentially "dead" and may leach minerals out of the body. However, it is highly effective against heavy metals.

Ionization is a means of adding negative ions to water to enable it to neutralize toxins (because they tend to have a positive electrical charge). Proponents claim that it renders the water more usable by the body's cells, allowing faster rehydration.

For specific brand recommendations and deals on some of my favorite water filtration systems, subscribe to my free e-zine, *World's Healthiest News*, at my site, www.DrMichelleCook.com.

Herb Suppliers

There are many excellent companies offering dried or bulk herbs that you may wish to use in your fermentation projects. Some of the herbs I've used in my fermented food recipes include licorice root (excellent for kombucha), green tea leaves (excellent for kombucha), cayenne chilies (great in pickled vegetable and sauerkraut recipes), juniper berries (excellent in sauerkraut), and, of course, the common culinary herbs like basil, oregano, rosemary, and others you might find tasty in your vegetable ferments. The companies include:

Aroma Borealis
www.aromaborealis.com

Harmonic Arts
www.harmonicarts.ca

Mountain Rose Herbs
www.mountainroseherbs.com

Diagnostic Tests

The following tests can help your physician determine whether you may have underlying microbial, nutritional, or neurotransmitter imbalances.

Nutra Eval by Genova/Metametrix measures 120 different compounds, including antioxidants, vitamins, neurotransmitters, dysbiosis, toxin levels, and essential fatty acids.

Genova/Metametrix, or Doctor's Data, gives a comprehensive stool analysis, including parasites and heavy-metal testing.

ZRT Labs has home test kits to assess 25-OH vitamin D levels.

Further Reading

Stephen Harrod Buhner. *Herbal Antibiotics: Natural Alternatives for Treating Drug-Resistant Bacteria*. North Adams, MA: Storey Publishing, 2012.

Michelle Schoffro Cook, PhD, ROHP. *Weekend Wonder Detox: Quick Cleanses to Strengthen Your Body and Enhance Your Beauty*. Boston: DaCapo Press, 2014.

Michelle Schoffro Cook, PhD, ROHP. *60 Seconds to Slim: Balance Your Body Chemistry to Burn Fat Fast!* Emmaus, PA: Rodale, 2013.

Jeff Cox. *The Essential Book of Fermentation: Great Taste and Good Health with Probiotic Foods*. New York: Avery, 2013.

Sandor Ellix Katz. *Wild Fermentation: The Flavor, Nutrition, and Craft of Live-Culture Foods*. White River Junction, VT: Chelsea Green, 2003.

Cobi Slater, PhD, DNM, RHT, RNCP. *The Ultimate Candida Guide and Cookbook: The Breakthrough Plan for Eliminating Disease-Causing Yeast and Revolutionizing Your Health!* Maitland, FL: Xulon Press, 2014.

Notes

Chapter 1: The Health Secret We've All Been Waiting For

1. Mary Ellen Sanders, "Probiotics: Definition, Selection, Sources, and Uses," *Clinical Infectious Diseases* 46, no. S2 (2008): S58–61. http://cid.oxfordjournals.org/content/46/Supplement_2/S58.full.

2. Stephen Harrod Buhner, *Herbal Antibiotics: Natural Alternatives for Treating Drug-Resistant Bacteria* (North Adams, MA: Storey Publishing, 2012), 44.

3. Hiromi Shinya, *The Microbe Factor: Your Innate Immunity and the Coming Health Revolution* (San Francisco: Council Oak Books, 2010), 28.

Chapter 2: The Surprising Worlds Within Your Body

1. Shinya, *The Microbe Factor*, 23.

2. Dan Krotz, "Berkeley Lab Scientists Help Define the Healthy Human Microbiome," Lawrence Berkeley National Laboratory, *News Center*, June 13, 2012, http://newscenter.lbl.gov/news-releases/2012/06/13/human-microbiome.

3. Jeff Cox, *The Essential Book of Fermentation: Great Taste and Good Health with Probiotic Foods* (New York: Avery, 2013), 39–40.

4. "Human Microbiome Project," National Institutes of Health, http://commonfund.nih.gov/hmp/index.

5. Donatella Comito, Antonio Cascio, and Claudio Romano, "Microbiota Biodiversity in Inflammatory Bowel Disease," *Italian Journal of Pediatrics* (March 31, 2014), www.ijponline.net/content/pdf/1824-7288-40-32.pdf.

6. Ibid.

7. Xandria Williams, *The Herbal Detox Plan: The Revolutionary Way to Cleanse and Revive Your Body* (Carlsbad, CA: Hay House, 2004), 83; Gloria Gilbere, "A Doctor's Solution to 'Plumbing Problems,' in Your Gut That Is!" *Total Health* 26, no. 1 (February 2004), 37.

8. Patricia Fitzgerald, *The Detox Solution: The Missing Link to Radiant Health, Abundant Energy, Ideal Weight, and Peace of Mind* (Santa Monica, CA: Illumination Press, 2001), 140.

9. Ibid.

10. Jacob Teitelbaum, *From Fatigued to Fantastic* (New York: Avery, 2007).

11. Cobi Slater, *The Ultimate Candida Guide and Cookbook: The Breakthrough Plan for Eliminating Disease-Causing Yeast and Revolutionizing Your Health!* (Maitland, FL: Xulon Press, 2014), 11.

12. Ibid., 16.

13. Michelle Schoffro Cook, *60 Seconds to Slim: Balance Your Body Chemistry to Burn Fat Fast!* (Emmaus, PA: Rodale, 2013), 184–188; Slater, *The Ultimate Candida Guide and Cookbook*, 16.

14. Cook, *60 Seconds to Slim*, 184–188.

15. "Vitamin," Oxford Dictionary, www.oxforddictionaries.com/definition /english/vitamin (emphasis added).

16. "Autoimmune Disorders," Medline Plus, www.nlm.nih.gov/medlineplus /ency/article/000816.htm.

17. Leonard Smith, "The Importance of Your Intestinal Tract for Health and Longevity," *Townsend Letter: The Examiner of Alternative Medicine*, April 2014, 70–72.

18. Emma J. Woodmansey, Marion E. T. McMurdo, George T. Macfarlane, and Sandra Macfarlane, "Comparison of Compositions and Metabolic Activities of Fecal Microbiotas in Young Adults and in Antibiotic-Treated and Non-Antibiotic-Treated Elderly Subjects," *Applied Environmental Microbiology* 10 (October 2007): 6113–6122.

19. Y. Guiqoz, J. Doré, and E. J. Schiffrin, "The Inflammatory Status of Old Age Can Be Nurtured from the Intestinal Environment," *Current Opinion in Clinical Nutrition and Metabolic Care* 11, no. 1 (January 2008): 13–20.

20. Smith, "The Importance of Your Intestinal Tract for Health and Longevity," 70.

21. Ibid.

22. Ibid.

23. M. A. Wozniak, A. L. Frost, and R. F. Itzhaki, "Alzheimer's Disease Specific Tau Phosphyloration Is Induced by Herpes Simplex Virus Type 1," *Journal of Alzheimer's Disease* 16, no. 2 (2009): 341–350; S. J. Soscia, et al., "The Alzheimer's Disease-Associated Amyloid Beta-Protein Is an Antimicrobial Peptide," *PLoS One* 5, no. 3 (March 2010): e9505.

24. L. A. David et al., "Diet Rapidly and Reproducibly Alters the Human Gut Microbiome," *Nature*, December 11, 2013, www.ncbi.nlm.nih.gov/ pubmed/24336217.

25. Michaeleen Doucleff, "Chowing Down on Meat, Dairy Alters Gut Bacteria a Lot, And Quickly," *NPR*, December 11, 2013, www.npr.org/blogs /thesalt/2013/12/10/250007042/chowing-down-on-meat-and-dairy-alters-gut -bacteria-a-lot-and-quickly.

26. K. Shinohara, Y. Ohashi, K. Kawasumi, A. Terada, and T. Fujisawa, "Effect of Apple Intake on Fecal Microbiota and Metabolites in Humans," *Anaerobe* 16, no. 5 (October 2010): 510–515, www.ncbi.nlm.nih.gov/pubmed /20304079.

Chapter 3: From the Common Cold to Superbugs: Probiotics to the Rescue

1. Buhner, *Herbal Antibiotics*, 26.

2. Ibid.

3. Brandon Keim, "Antibiotics Breed Superbugs Faster Than Expected," Wired.com, December 22, 2010.

4. Chris Wodskou, "Bacteria Getting Upper Hand in Antibiotics Arms Race," *CBC News*, March 1, 2014, www.cbc.ca/news/health/bacteria-getting -upper-hand-in-antibiotics-arms-race-1.2555750.

5. Buhner, *Herbal Antibiotics*, 17.

6. Ibid., 18.

7. Ibid., 19.

8. Ibid.

9. Stuart B. Levy, *The Antibiotic Paradox: How the Misuse of Antibiotics Destroys Their Curative Power* (New York: Plenum Press, 1992), 94.

10. "Antibiotic Resistance Threats in the US," Centers for Disease Control and Prevention, www.cdc.gov/features/AntibioticResistanceThreats/index.html.

11. Buhner, *Herbal Antibiotics*, 40.

12. Ibid.

13. Ibid., 27–28.

14. Philip Hilts, "Gene Jumps to Spread a Toxin in Meat," *New York Times*, April 23, 1996, www.nytimes.com/1996/04/23/science/gene-jumps-to-spread-a -toxin-in-meat.html.

15. Buhner, *Herbal Antibiotics*, 31.

16. Wodskou, "Bacteria Getting Upper Hand in Antibiotics Arms Race."

17. Y. Qin, J. Li, Q. Wang, K. Gao, B. Zhu, and N. Lv, "Identification of Lactic Acid Bacteria in Commercial Yogurt and Their Antibiotic Resistance," *Wei Sheng Wu Xue Bao* 53, no. 8 (August 4, 2013): 897, www.ncbi.nlm.nih .gov/pubmed/24341282.

18. Mary Ellen Sanders, "How Do We Know When Something Called "Probiotic" Is Really a Probiotic? A Guideline for Consumers and Health Care Professionals," *Functional Food Reviews* 1, no. 1 (Spring 2009): 3–12.

19. A. Lyra et al., "Comparison of Bacterial Quantities in Left and Right Colon Biopsies and Faeces," *World Journal of Gastroenterology* 18, no. 32 (August 28, 2012): 4404–4411, www.ncbi.nlm.nih.gov/pubmed/22969206.

20. X. W. Gao, M. Mubasher, C. Y. Fang, C. Reifer, and L. E. Miller, "Dose Response Efficacy of a Proprietary Probiotic Formula of *Lactobacillus acidophilus CL1285* and *Lactobacillus casei LBC80R* for Antibiotic-Associated Diarrhea and *Clostridium difficile*-Associated Diarrhea Prophylaxis in Adult Patients," *American Journal of Gastroenterology* 105, no. 7 (July 2010): 1636–1641, www.ncbi.nlm.nih.gov/pubmed/20145608.

21. E. J. Videlock and F. Cremonini, "Meta-Analysis: Probiotics in Antibiotic-Associated Diarrhea," *Alimentary Pharmacology and Therapeutics* 35, no. 12 (June 2012): 1355–1369, www.ncbi.nlm.nih.gov/pubmed/22531096.

22. E. Lönnermark, V. Friman, G. Lappas, T. Sandberg, A. Berggren, and I. Adlerberth, "Intake of *Lactobacillus plantarum* Reduces Certain Gastrointestinal Symptoms During Treatment with Antibiotics," *Journal of Clinical Gastroenterology* 44, no. 2 (February 2010): 106–112, www.ncbi.nlm.nih.gov /pubmed/19727002.

23. M. Hickson, A. I. D'Souza, N. Muthu, T. R. Rogers, S. Want, C. Rajkumar, and C. J. Bulpitt, "Use of Probiotic *Lactobacillus* Preparation to Prevent Diarrhoea Associated with Antibiotics: Randomised Double Blind Placebo Controlled Trial," *BMJ: Clinical Research Edition* 335, no. 7612 (July 2007), www.ncbi.nlm.nih.gov/pubmed/1914504.

24. "Product Review: Probiotics for Adults, Children, and Pets," ConsumerLab.com, November 23, 2013, www.consumberlab.com/results/print .asp?reviewid=probiotics.

25. Ibid.

26. "Diseases and Conditions: Periodontitis," Mayo Clinic, www.mayo clinic.org/diseases-conditions/periodontitis/basics/definition/con-20021679.

27. W. Teughels, A. Durukan, O. Ozcelik, M. Pauwels, M. Quirynen, and M. C. Haytac, "Clinical and Microbiological Effects of *Lactobacillus reuteri* Probiotics in the Treatment of Chronic Periodontitis: A Randomized Placebo-Controlled Study," *Journal of Clinical Periodontitis* 40, no. 11 (November 2013): 1025–1035, www.ncbi.nlm.nih.gov/pubmed/24164569.

28. "What Is Peptic Ulcer Disease?" WebMD, www.webmd.com/digestive -disorders/digestive-diseases-peptic-ulcer-disease.

29. "What Is Gastritis?" WebMD, www.webmd.com/digestive-disorders /digestive-diseases-gastritis.

30. E. P. Iakovenko et al., "Effects of Probiotic Bifiform on Efficacy of *Helicobacter pylori* Infection Treatment," *Terapevticheskii rkhiv* 78, no. 2 (2006): 21–26, www.ncbi.nlm.nih.gov/pubmed/16613091.

31. Ibid.

32. "Product Review: Probiotics for Adults, Children, and Pets."

33. Lucia Pacifico et al., "Probiotics for the Treatment of *Helicobacter pylori* Infection in Children," *World Journal of Gastroenterology* 20, no. 3 (January 21, 2014): 673–683, www.ncbi.nlm.nih.gov/pmc/articles/PMC3921477.

34. Y. Aiba, N. Suzuki, A. M. Kabir, A. Takagi, and Y. Koga, "Lactic Acid-Mediated Suppression of *Helicobacter pylori* by the Oral Administration of *Lactobacillus salivarius* as a Probiotic in a Gnotobiotic Murine Model," *American Journal of Gastroenterology* 93, no. 11 (1998): 2097–2101, www .ncbi.nlm.nih.gov/pubmed/9820379; M. H. Coconnier, V. Lievin, E. Hemery, and A. L. Servin, "Antagonistic Activity Against *Helicobacter* Infection in Vitro and in Vivo by the Human *Lactobacillus acidophilus* Strain *LB*," *Applied Environmental Microbiology* 64, no. 11 (1998): 4573–4580, www.ncbi.nlm .nih.gov/pubmed/9797324; K. C. Johnson-Henry, D. J. Mitchell, Y. Avitzur, E. Galindo-Mata, N. L. Jones, and P. M. Sherman, "Probiotics Reduce Bacterial Colonization and Gastric Inflammation in *H. pylori*-Infected Mice," *Digestive Diseases and Sciences* 49, no. 7–8 (2004): 1095–1102, www.ncbi.nlm.nih. gov/pubmed/15387328; A. M. Kabir, Y. Aiba, A. Takagi, S. Kamiya, T. Miwa, and Y. Koga, "Prevention of *Helicobacter pylori* Infection by Lactobacilli in a Gnotobiotic Murine Model," *Gut* 41, no. 9707 (1997): 49–55, www.ncbi .nlm.nih.gov/pubmed/9274471; D. N. Sgouras, E. G. Panayotopoulou, B. Martinez-Gonzalez, K. Petraki, S. Michopoulos, and A. Mentis, "*Lactobacillus johnsonii La1* Attenuates *Helicobacter pylori*-Associated Gastritis and Reduces Levels of Proinflammatory Chemokines in C57BL/6 Mice," *Clinical and Diagnostic Laboratory Immunology* 12, no. 12 (2005): 1378–1386, www.ncbi.nlm .nih.gov/pubmed/16339060.

35. M. Gotteland et al., "Modulation of *Helicobacter pylori* Colonization with Cranberry Juice and *Lactobacillus johnsonii La1* in Children," *Nutrition* 24, no. 5 (2008): 421–426, www.ncbi.nlm.nih.gov/pubmed/18343637.

36. Pacifico et al., "Probiotics for the Treatment of *Helicobacter pylori* Infection in Children."

37. H. Sikorska and W. Smoragiewica, "Role of Probiotics in the Prevention and Treatment of Methicillin-Resistant *Staphylococcus aureus* Infections," *International Journal of Antimicrobial Agents* 42, no. 6 (December 2013): 475–481, www.ncbi.nlm.nih.gov/pubmed/24071026.

38. P.-W. Chen, T. T. Jheng, C.-L. Shyu, and F. C. Mao, "Synergistic Antibacterial Efficacies of the Combination of Bovine Lactoferrin or its Hydrolysate

with Probiotic Secretion in Curbing the Growth of Meticillin-Resistant *Staphylococcus aureus*," *Journal of Medical Microbiology* 62, no. 12 (December 2013): 1845–1851, www.ncbi.nlm.nih.gov/pubmed/24072764.

39. C. R. Musgrave, P. B. Bookstaver, S. S. Sutton, and A. D. Miller, "Use of Alternative or Adjuvant Pharmacologic Treatment Strategies in the Prevention and Treatment of *Clostridium difficile* Infection," *International Journal of Infectious Disease* 15, no. 7 (July 2012): 3438–448, www.ncbi.nlm.nih.gov/pubmed /21596604.

40. B. A. Haywood, Katherine E. Black, Dane Baker, James McGarvey, Phil Healey, and Rachel C. Brown, "Probiotic Supplementation Reduces the Duration and Incidence of Infections but Not Severity in Elite Rugby Union Players," *Journal of Science and Medicine in Sport* 17, no. 4 (August 31, 2013): 356–360, www.ncbi.nlm.nih.gov/pubmed/?term=j+sci+med+sport+probiotics.

41. M. Popova et al., "Beneficial Effects of Probiotics in Upper Respiratory Tract Infections and Their Mechanical Actions to Antagonize Pathogens," *Journal of Applied Microbiology* 113, no. 6 (July 2012): 1305–1318, www .ncbi.nlm.nih.gov/pubmed/22788970.

42. R. Luoto, O. Ruuskanen, M. Waris, M. Kalliomäki, S. Salminen, and E. Isolauri, "Prebiotic and Probiotic Supplementation Prevents Rhinovirus Infections in Preterm Infants," *Journal of Allergy and Clinical Immunology* 133, no. 2 (October 13, 2013): 405–413, www.ncbi.nlm.nih.gov/pubmed/24131826.

43. E. Guillemard, F. Tondu, F. Lacoin, and J. Schrezenmeir, "Consumption of a Fermented Dairy Product Containing the Probiotic *Lactobacillus casei DN-114001* Reduces the Duration of Respiratory Infections in the Elderly in a Randomised Controlled Trial," *British Journal of Nutrition* 103, no. 1 (January 2010): 58–68, www.ncbi.nlm.nih.gov/pubmed/19747410.

44. John Heinerman, *Heinerman's Encyclopedia of Healing Herbs and Spices* (New York: Reward Books, 1996), 333.

45. P. Mastromarino, Fatima Cacciotti, Alessandra Masci, and Luciana Mosca, "Antiviral Activity of *Lactobacillus brevis* Towards Herpes Simplex Virus Type 2: Role of Cell Wall Associated Components," *Anaerobe* 17, no. 6 (December 2011): 334–336, www.ncbi.nlm.nih.gov/pubmed/21621625.

46. E. I. Ermolenko, V. A. Furaeva, V. A. Isakov, D. K. Ermolenko, and A. N. Survorov, "Inhibition of Herpes Simplex Virus Type 1 Reproduction by Probiotic Bacteria in Vitro," *Voprosy Virusologii* 55, no. 4 (July–August 2010): 25–28, www.ncbi.nlm.nih.gov/pubmed/20886709.

47. T. M. Liaskovs'kyi, S. L. Rybalko, V. S. Pidhors'kyi, N. K. Kovalenko, and L. T. Oleshchenko, "Effect of Probiotic Lactic Acid Bacteria Strains on

Virus Infection," *Mikrobiolohichnyi zhurnal* 69, no. 2 (March/April 2007): 55–63, www.ncbi.nlm.nih.gov/pubmed/17494336.

48. C. Rask, I. Adlerberth, A. Berggren, I. L. Ahrén, and A. E. Wold, "Differential Effect on Cell-Mediated Immunity in Human Volunteers After Intake of Different Lactobacilli," *Clinical and Experimental Immunology* 172, no. (May 2013): 321–332, www.ncbi.nlm.nih.gov/pubmed/23574328.

49. Ananya Mandal, "What Is a Macrophage?" *News Medical*, www.news-medical.net/health/What-is-a-Macrophage.aspx.

50. "Worldwide AIDS and HIV Statistics," AVERT, www.avert.org/world stats.htm.

51. M. I. Petrova, M. van den Broek, J. Vanderleyden, S. Lebeer, and J. Balzarini, "Vaginal Microbiota and Its Role in HIV Transmission and Infection," *FEMS Microbiology Review* 37, no. 5 (September 2013): 762–792, www.ncbi.nlm.nih.gov/pubmed/23789590.

52. Neetu Gautam et al., "Role of Multivitamins, Micronutrients and Probiotics Supplementation in Management of HIV Infected Children," *Indian Journal of Pediatrics* (April 24, 2014), www.ncbi.nlm.nih.gov/pubmed/24760382.

53. H. Hu et al., "Impact of Eating Probiotic Yogurt on Colonization by Candida Species of the Oral and Vaginal Mucosa in HIV-Infected and HIV-Uninfected Women," *Mycopathologia* 176, no. 3–4 (October 2013): 175–181, www.ncbi.nlm.nih.gov/pubmed/23925786.

54. G. Reid et al., "Oral Use of *Lactobacillus rhamnosus GR-1* and *L. fermentum RC-14* Significantly Alters Vaginal Flora: Randomized, Placebo-Controlled Trial in 64 Healthy Women," *FEMS Immunology and Medical Microbiology* 35, no. 2 (March 20, 2003): 131–134, www.ncbi.nlm.nih.gov/pubmed/12628548.

55. Cook, *60 Seconds to Slim*, 184–188.

56. H. B. Wang, "Cellulase Assisted Extraction and Antibacterial Activity of Polysaccharides from the Dandelion Taraxacum Officinale," *Carbohydrate Polymers* 103 (March 15, 2014): 140–142, www.ncbi.nlm.nih.gov/pubmed/24528711.

57. O.-H. Lee and B.-Y. Lee, "Antioxidant and Antimicrobial Activities of Individual and Combined Phenolics in Olea Europaea Leaf Extract," *Bioresource Technology* 101, no. 10 (May 2010): 3751–3754, www.ncbi.nlm.nih.gov/pubmed/ 20106659.

58. Michelle Schoffro Cook, "4 Natural Antibiotics," Care2, November 30, 2011, www.care2.com/greenliving/4-natural-antibiotics.html.

Chapter 4: New Hope for Serious Illnesses

1. Brian Krans, "Mood Disorders Linked to Inflammation," *Healthline News*, June 12, 2013, www.healthline.com/health-news/mental-mood-disorders -tied-to-autoimmune-diseases-infection-061213.

2. Artemis Morris and Molly Rossiter, "Linking Inflammation to Chronic Diseases," For Dummies, www.dummies.com/how-to/content/linking -inflammation-to-chronic-diseases.html.

3. Ibid.

4. Ibid.

5. David M. Marquis, "Inflammation Affects Every Aspect of Your Health," Mercola, March 7, 2013, http://articles.mercola.com/sites/articles/archive /2013/03/07/inflammation-triggers-disease-symptoms.aspx.

6. Ibid.

7. Ibid.

8. Ibid.

9. Carmen Rondon and Cemal Cingi, "Allergic Rhinoconjunctivitis," EAACI, http://infoallergy.com/Tools-Extras/Allergic-Rhinoconjunctivitis.

10. M. Tamura et al., "Effects of Probiotics on Allergic Rhinitis Induced by Japanese Cedar Pollen: Randomized Double-Blind, Placebo-Controlled Clinical Trial," *International Archives of Allergy and Immunology* 143, no 1 (December 2007): 75–82, www.ncbi.nlm.nih.gov/pubmed/17199093.

11. M. A. Moyad et al., "Immunogenic Yeast-Based Fermentation Product Reduces Allergic Rhinitis-Induced Nasal Congestion: A Randomized, Double-Blind, Placebo-Controlled Trial," *Advanced Therapeutics* 26, no. 8 (2009): 795–804.

12. "Facts and Statistics," Anxiety and Depression Association of America, www.adaa.org/about-adaa/press-room/facts-statistics.

13. ConsumerLab.com, "Product Review: Probiotics for Adults, Children and Pets."

14. P. Bercik et al., "Chronic Gastrointestinal Inflammation Induces Anxiety-Like Behavior and Alters Central Nervous System Biochemistry in Mice," *Gastroenterology* 139, no. 6 (December 2010): 2102–2112, www.ncbi.nlm.nih.gov /pubmed/20600016.

15. Ibid.

16. J. Fehér, I. Kovács, and C. Balacco Gabrieli, "Role of Gastrointestinal Inflammations in the Development and Treatment of Depression," *Orvosi Hetilap* 152, no. 37 (September 2011): 1477–1485, www.ncbi.nlm.nih.gov/pubmed /21893478.

17. M. Messaoudi et al., "Assessment of Psychotropic-Like Properties of a Probiotic Formulation (*Lactobacillus helveticus R0052* and *Bifidobacterium longum R0175*) in Rats and Human Subjects," *British Journal of Nutrition* 105, no. 5 (March 2011): 755–764, www.ncbi.nlm.nih.gov/pubmed/20974015.

18. L. Pineda Mde, S. F. Thompson, K. Summers, F. de Leon, J. Pope, and G. Reid, "A Randomized, Double-Blind, Placebo-Controlled Pilot Study of Probiotics in Active Rheumatoid Arthritis," *Medical Science Monitor* 17, no. 6 (June 2011): CR347–354, www.ncbi.nlm.nih.gov/pubmed?term=rheumatoid%20arthritis%20university%20of%20western%20probiotic.

19. Nina Lincoff, "Gut Bacteria May Cause Inflammation in Rheumatoid Arthritis," *HealthlineNews*, November 8, 2013, www.healthline.com/health-news/arthritis-gut-bacteria-may-trigger-ra-110813.

20. Michelle Schoffro Cook, *The Brain Wash* (Toronto, Ontario: John Wiley and Sons, 2007), 2.

21. Guillemard, Tondu, Lacoin, and Schrezenmeir, "Consumption of a Fermented Dairy Product Containing the Probiotic *Lactobacillus casei DN114001* Reduces the Duration of Respiratory Infections in the Elderly in a Randomised Controlled Trial."

22. Alan C. Logan, *The Brain Diet: The Connection Between Nutrition, Mental Health, and Intelligence* (Nashville, TN: Cumberland House Publishing, 2006), 115.

23. National Cancer Institute, "Surveillance, Epidemiology, and End Results Program: Turning Cancer Data into Discovery," http://seer.cancer.gov/statfacts/html/all.html.

24. T. Ohara, K. Yoshino, and M. Kitajima, "Possibility of Preventing Colorectal Carcinogenesis with Probiotics," *Hepatogastroenterology* 57, no. 104 (November–December 2010): 1411–1415, www.ncbi.nlm.nih.gov/pubmed/21443095.

25. M. Reale et al., "Daily Intake of *Lactobacillus casei Shirota* Increases Natural Killer Cell Activity in Smokers," *British Journal of Nutrition* 108, no. 2 (July 2012): 308–314, www.ncbi.nlm.nih.gov/pubmed/22142891.

26. P. D. Cani, M. Osto, L. Geurts, and A. Everard, "Involvement of Gut Microbiota in the Development of Low Grade Inflammation and Type 2 Diabetes Associated with Diabetes," *Gut Microbes* 3, no. 4 (July 2012): 279–288, www.ncbi.nlm.nih.gov/pubmed/22572877.

27. Z. Asemi, Z. Zare, H. Shakeri, S. S. Sabihi, and A. Esmaillzadeh, "Effect of Multispecies Probiotic Supplements on Metabolic Profiles, hs-CRP, and Oxidative Stress in Patients with Type 2 Diabetes," *Annals of Nutrition and Metabolism* 63, no. 1–2 (July 5, 2013): 1–9, www.ncbi.nlm.nih.gov/pubmed/23899653.

28. Bruno Melo Carvalho and Mario Jose Abdalla Saad, "Influence of Gut Microbiota on Subclinical Inflammation and Insulin Resistance," *Mediators of Inflammation* 2013, 6778 (2013): 1–13, www.ncbi.nlm.nih.gov/pubmed /23840101.

29. P. Bekkering, I. Jafri, F. J. Overveld, and G. T. Rijkers, "The Intricate Association Between Gut Microbiota and Development of Type 1, Type 2 and Type 3 Diabetes," *Expert Reviews in Clinical Immunology* 9, no. 11 (November 2013): 1031–1041, www.ncbi.nlm.nih.gov/pubmed/24138599.

30. R. D'Arienzo et al., "Immunomodulatory Effects of *Lactobacillus casei* Administration in a Mouse Model of Gliaden-Sensitive Enteropathy," *Scandinavian Journal of Immunology* 74, no. 4 (October 2011): 3335–3341, www .ncbi.nlm.nih.gov/pubmed/21615450.

31. Michelle Schoffro Cook, *The Phytozyme Cure* (Toronto, Ontario: Wiley and Sons, 2010), 179.

32. Mark W. Hull and Paul L. Beck, "*Clostridium difficile*-Associated Colitis," *Canadian Family Physician* 50 (November 2004): 1536–1545, www.ncbi .nlm.nih.gov/pubmed/15597970.

33. Donatella Comito, Antonio Cascio, and Claudio Romano, "Microbiota Biodiversity in Inflammatory Bowel Disease," *Italian Journal of Pediatrics* 40, no. 1 (March 31, 2014): 32, www.ncbi.nlm.nih.gov/pubmed/24684926.

34. "Diseases and Conditions: Irritable Bowel Syndrome—Definition," Mayo Clinic, www.mayoclinic.org/diseases-conditions/irritable-bowel-syndrome /basics/definition/con-20024578.

35. Ibid.

36. P. J. Whorwell, "Review: Do Probiotics Improve Symptoms in Patients with Irritable Bowel Syndrome?" *Therapeutic Advances in Gastroenterology* 2, no. S4 (July 2009): S37–S34, www.ncbi.nlm.nih.gov/pubmed/21180553.

37. F. Indrio et al., "Prophylactic Use of a Probiotic in the Prevention of Colic, Regurgitation, and Functional Constipation: A Randomized Clinical Trial," *JAMA Pediatrics* 168, no. 3 (March 1, 2014): 228–233, www.ncbi.nlm .nih.gov/pubmed/24424513.

38. P. J. Whorwell et al., "Efficacy of an Encapsulated Probiotic *Bifidobacterium infantis 35624* in Women with Irritable Bowel Syndrome," *American Journal of Gastroenterology* 101, no. 7 (July 2006): 1581–1590, www.ncbi .nlm.nih.gov/pubmed/16863564.

39. H. J. Kim et al., "A Randomized Controlled Trial of a Probiotic Combination VSL#3 and Placebo in Irritable Bowel Syndrome with Bloating," *Neurogastroenterology and Motility* 17, no. 5 (October 2005): 687–696, www.ncbi .nlm.nih.gov/pubmed/16185307.

40. B. Ki Cha et al., "The Effect of a Multispecies Probiotic Mixture on the Symptoms and Fecal Microbiota in Diarrhea-Dominant Irritable Bowel Syndrome: A Randomized, Double-Blind, Placebo-Controlled Trial," *Journal of Clinical Gastroenterology* 46, no. 3 (March 2012): 220–227, www.ncbi .nlm.nih.gov/pubmed/22157240.

41. D. H. Sinn et al., "Therapeutic Effect of *Lactobacillus acidophilus-SDC 2012, 2013* in Patients with Irritable Bowel Syndrome," *Digestive Diseases and Sciences* 53, no. 10 (October 2008): 2714–2718, www.ncbi.nlm.nih.gov /pubmed/18274900.

42. Claudio Romano et al., "*Lactobacillus reuteri* in Children with Functional Abdominal Pain (FAP)," *Journal of Pediatrics and Child Health* 9 (July 8, 2010), www.ncbi.nlm.nih.gov/pubmed/20626584.

43. Whorwell, "Review: Do Probiotics Improve Symptoms in Patients with Irritable Bowel Syndrome?"

44. A. Tursi et al., "Randomised Clinical Trial: Mesalazine and/or Probiotics in Maintaining Remission of Symptomatic Uncomplicated Diverticular Disease—A Double-Blind, Randomised, Placebo-Controlled Study," *Alimentary Pharmacology and Therapeutics* 38, no. 7 (October 2013): 741–751, www .ncbi.nlm.nih.gov/pubmed/23957734.

45. Kenneth D. Kochanek, Jaquan Xu, Sherry L. Murphy, Arialdi M. Miniño, and Hsiang-Ching Kung, "Deaths: Final Data for 2009," *National Vital Statistics Reports* 60, no. 3 (2011), www.cdc.gov/nchs/data/nvsr/nvsr60/nvsr60_03.pdf.

46. D. B. DiRienzo, "Effects of Probiotics on Biomarkers of Cardiovascular Disease: Implications for Heart-Healthy Diets," *Nutrition Reviews* 72, no. 1 (January 2014): 18–29, www.ncbi.nlm.nih.gov/pubmed/24330093.

47. R. Ben Salah, I. Trabelsi, K. Hamden, H. Chouayekh, and S. Bejar, "*Lactobacillus plantarum TN8* Exhibits Protective Effects on Lipid, Hepatic and Renal Profiles in Obese Rats," *Anaerobe* 23 (October 2013): 55–61, www.ncbi .nlm.nih.gov/pubmed/23891961.

48. P. Hlivak, J. Odraska, M. Ferencki, L. Ebringer, E. Jahnova, and Z. Mikes, "One-Year Application of Probiotic Strain *Enterococcus faecium M-74* Decreases in Serum Cholesterol Levels," *Bratislavske Lekarske Listy* 106, no. 2 (2005): 67–72, www.ncbi.nlm.nih.gov/pubmed/16026136.

49. M. L. Jones, C. J. Martoni, and S. Prakash, "Cholesterol Lowering and Inhibition of Sterol Absorption by *Lactobacillus reuteri NCIMB 30242*: A Randomized Controlled Trial," *European Journal of Clinical Nutrition* 66, no. 11 (November 2012): 1234–1241, www.ncbi.nlm.nih.gov/22990854.

50. Medline Plus, "C-Reactive Protein," www.nlm.nih.gov/medlineplus/ency /article/003356.htm.

51. U. Hoppu, Erika Isolauri, Pèaivi Laakso, Jaakko Matomèaki, and Kirso Laitinen, "Probiotics and Dietary Counselling Targeting Maternal Dietary Fat Intake Modifies Breast Milk Fatty Acids and Cytokines," *European Journal of Nutrition* 51, no. 2 (March 2012): 211–219, www.ncbi.nlm.nih.gov/pubmed/21626296.

52. Logan, *The Brain Diet*, 114.

Chapter 5: How to Select Probiotic Supplements

1. Logan, *The Brain Diet*, 114.

2. "The Probiotic Leader: Functions of Probiotic Species," Klaire Labs, www.klaire.com/probioticleader3.htm.

3. Ibid.

4. Ibid.

5. Ibid.

6. "*C. difficile* Infection," Mayo Clinic, www.mayoclinic.org/diseases-conditions/c-difficile/basics/definition/con-20029664.

7. "Listeria," Microbe Wiki, http://microbewiki.kenyon.edu/index.php/Listeria.

8. "Enterococcus," Microbe Wiki, http://microbewiki.kenyon.edu/index.php/Enterococcus.

9. "MRSA Infection," Mayo Clinic, www.mayoclinic.org/diseases-conditions/mrsa/basics/definition/CON-20024479.

10. "The Probiotic Leader: Functions of Probiotic Species."

11. Ibid.

12. Ibid.

13. "*Salmonella typhimurium*," Microbe Wiki, http://microbewiki.kenyon.edu/index.php/Salmonella_typhimurium.

14. "*Bifidobacterium*," Wikipedia, http://en.wikipedia.org/wiki/Bifidobacterium.

15. "The Probiotic Leader: Functions of Probiotic Species."

16. Ibid.

17. "*Bacteroides*," Microbe Wiki, http://microbewiki.kenyon.edu/index.php/Bacteroides.

18. "*Campylobacter jejuni*," Microbe Wiki, http://microbewiki.kenyon.edu/index.php/Campylobacter_jejuni; Microbe Wiki, "Rotavirus," http://microbewiki.kenyon.edu/index.php/Rotavirus.

19. "The Probiotic Leader: Functions of Probiotic Species."

20. Ibid.

21. Ibid.

22. Ibid.

23. Deirdre Rawlings, *Fermented Foods for Health: Use the Power of Probiotic Foods to Improve Your Digestion, Strengthen Your Immunity, and Prevent Illness* (Beverly, MA: Fair Winds Press, 2013), 13.

24. "The Probiotic Leader: Functions of Probiotic Species."

25. "Product Review: Probiotics for Adults, Children and Pets."

26. "*Lactobacillus*—Interactions," WebMD, www.webmd.com/vitamins-supplements/ingredientmono-790-lactobacillus.aspx?activeingredientid=790&activeingredientname=lactobacillus.

27. "Product Review: Probiotics for Adults, Children and Pets."

28. Ibid.

29. Ibid.

30. Ibid.

Chapter 6: Fall in Love with Fermented Foods

1. Rawlings, *Fermented Foods for Health*, 5.

2. Ibid.

3. Fabíola Málaga Barreto et al., "Beneficial Effects of *Lactobacillus plantarum* on Glycemia and Homocysteine Levels in Postmenopausal Women with Metabolic Syndrome," *Nutrition* 30, no. 7–8 (December 14, 2013): 939–942, www.ncbi.nlm.nih.gov/pubmed/24613434.

4. "Diseases and Conditions: Metabolic Syndrome," Mayo Clinic, www.mayoclinic.org/diseases-conditions/metabolic-syndrome/basics/definition/con-20027243.

5. Patrick Holford, *The New Optimum Nutrition Bible: Revised and Updated* (Berkeley, CA: Crossing Press, 2004), 137, 139.

6. Guillemard, Tondu, Lacoin, and Schrezenmeir, "Consumption of a Fermented Dairy Product Containing the Probiotic *Lactobacillus casei DN-114001* Reduces the Duration of Respiratory Infections in the Elderly in a Randomised Controlled Trial."

7. "Your Health in Postmenopause," WebMD, www.webmd.com/menopause/guide/health-after-menopause.

8. F. Aragon, G. Perdigon, A. De Moreno de LeBlanc, and S. Carino, "The Administration of Milk Fermented by the Probiotic *Lactobacillus casei CRL 431* Exerts an Immunomodulatory Effect Against a Breast Tumour in a Mouse

Model," *Immunobiology* 219, no. 6 (February 25, 2014): 457–464, www.ncbi
.nlm.nih.gov/pubmed/24646876.

9. Aarti Sachdeva, Swapnil Rawat, and J. Nagpal, "Efficacy of Fermented
Milk and Whey Proteins in *Helicobacter pylori* Eradication: A Review," *World
Journal of Gastroenterology* 20, no. 3 (January 21, 2014): 724–737, www.ncbi
.nlm.nih.gov/pubmed/24574746.

10. Ibid.

11. E. Zagato et al., "*Lactobacillus paracasei CBA L74* Metabolic Products
and Fermented Milk for Infant Formula Have Anti-Inflammatory Activity on
Dendritic Cells in Vitro and Protective Effects Against Colitis and an Enteric
Pathogen in Vivo," *PLoS One* 9, no. 2 (February 10, 2014): e87615, www.ncbi
.nlm.nih.gov/pubmed/24520333.

12. Kazuhito Ohsawa, Naoto Uchida, Kohji Ohki, Yasunori Nakamura,
and Hidehiko Yokogoshi, "*Lactobacillus helveticus*-Fermented Milk Improves
Learning and Memory in Mice," *Nutritional Neuroscience* (April 3, 2014),
www.ncbi.nlm.nih.gov/pubmed/24694020.

13. Michelle Schoffro Cook, *Weekend Wonder Detox: Quick Cleanses to
Strengthen Your Body and Enhance Your Beauty* (Boston: Da Capo Press,
2014).

14. H. Kikuchi-Hayakawa et al., "Effects of Soy Milk and Bifidobacterium
Fermented Soy Milk on Lipid Metabolism in Aged Ovariectomized Rats," *Bio-
science, Biotechnology, and Biochemistry* 62, no. 9 (September 1998): 1688–
1692, www.ncbi.nlm.nih.gov/pubmed/9805369.

15. Y. A. Sinyavsky, V. A. Kraysman, and Zh. M. Sulymenova, "Using of a Specialized Fermented Milk Product on the Basis of Soybeans in Cardiology Practice," *Voprosy Pitaniia* 82, no. 5 (2013): 51–57, www.ncbi.nlm.nih.gov/pubmed
/24640160.

16. C. P. Cheng, S. W. Tsai, C. P. Chiu, T. M. Pan, and T. Y Tsai, "The Effect
of Probiotic-Fermented Soy Milk on Enhancing the NO-Mediated Vascular
Relaxation Factors," *Journal of Science and Food Agriculture* 93, no. 5 (March
30, 2013): 1219–1225, www.ncbi.nlm.nih.gov/pubmed/22996620.

17. Li-Ru Lai, Shu-Chen Hsieh, and Hui-Yu Huang, "Effect of Lactic Fermentation on the Total Phenolic, Saponin, and Phytic Acid Contents as Well as
Anti-Colon Cancer Cell Proliferation Activity of Soymilk," *Journal of Biosci-
ence and Bioengineering* 115, no. 5 (May 2013): 552–556, www.ncbi.nlm.nih
.gov/pubmed/23290992.

18. S. K. Yeo and M. T. Liong, "Angiotensin I-Converting Enzyme Inhibi-
tory Activity and Bioconversion of Isoflavones by Probiotics in Soymilk Supplemented with Prebiotics," *International Journal of Food Science Nutrition* 61,
no. 2 (March 2010): 161–181, www.ncbi.nlm.nih.gov/pubmed/20085504.

19. Michelle Schoffro Cook, *The Phytozyme Cure: Treat or Reverse More Than 30 Serious Health Conditions with Powerful Plant Nutrients* (Toronto, Ontario: John Wiley and Sons, 2010), 220–221.

20. S. M. Lee, Y. Kim, H. J. Choi, J. Choi, Y. Yi, and S. Yoon, "Soy Milk Suppresses Cholesterol-Induced Inflammatory Gene Expression and Improves the Fatty Acid Profile in the Skin of SD Rats," *Biochemical and Biophysical Research Communications* 430, no. 1 (January 4, 2013): 202–207, www.ncbi .nlm.nih.gov/pubmed/23111331.

21. K. Miyazaki, T. Hanamizu, T. Sone, K. Chiba, T. Kinoshita, and S. Yoshikawa, "Topical Application of Bifidobacterium-Fermented Soy Milk Extract Containing Genistein and Daidzein Improves Rheological and Physiological Properties of Skin," *Journal of Cosmetic Sciences* 55, no. 5 (September/October 2004): 473–479, www.ncbi.nlm.nih.gov/pubmed/15608997.

22. S. Inoguchi, Y. Ohashi, A. Narai-Kanayama, K. Aso, T. Makagaki, and T. Fujisawa, "Effects of Non-Fermented and Fermented Soybean Milk Intake on Faecal Microbiota and Faecal Metabolites in Humans," *International Journal of Food Science and Nutrition* 63, no. 4 (June 2012): 402–410, www.ncbi .nlm.nih.gov/pubmed/22040525.

23. "Genistein," Phytochemicals.info, www.phytochemicals.info/phyto chemicals/genistein.php.

24. Ibid.

25. Lai, Hsieh, and Huang, "Effect of Lactic Fermentation on the Total Phenolic, Saponin, and Phytic Acid Contents as Well as Anti-Colon Cancer Cell Proliferation Activity of Soymilk."

26. Takuya Sato, Yasutomo Shinohara, Daisuke Kaneko, Ikuko Nishimura, and Asahi Matsuyama, "Fermented Soymilk Increases Voluntary Wheel Running Activity and Sexual Behavior in Male Rats," *Applied Physiology, Nutrition, and Metabolism* 35, no. 6 (December 2010): 749–754, www.ncbi.nlm.nih .gov/pubmed/21164545.

27. Terri Coles, "Kefir Benefits: 12 Things to Know About This Yogurt-Like Food," *Huffington Post*, September 12, 2013, www.huffingtonpost.ca/2013/09 /12/kefir-benefits_n_3914818.html.

28. Terri Coles, "Kefir Benefits: 12 Things to Know About This Yogurt-Like Food," *Huffington Post*, September 12, 2013, http://www.huffingtonpost.ca /2013/09/12/kefir-benefits_n_3914818.html.

29. Ibid.; Cox, *The Essential Book of Fermentation*, 21.

30. H. Maeda, X. Zhu, K. Omura, S. Suzuki, and S. Kitamura, "Effects of an Exopolysaccharide (kefiran) on Lipids, Blood Pressure, Blood Glucose, and Constipation," *Biofactors* 22, no. 1–4 (2004): 197–200, www.ncbi.nlm.nih.gov /pubmed/15630283.

31. A. M. de Oliveira Leite, J. T. Silva, V. M. F. Paschoalin, M. A. L. Miguel, R. S. Peixoto, and A. S. Rosado, "Microbiological, Technological, and Therapeutic Properties of Kefir: A Natural Probiotic Beverage," *Brazilian Journal of Microbiology* 44, no. 2 (October 30, 2013): 341–349, www.ncbi.nlm.nih.gov/pubmed/24294220.

32. Y. P. Chen and M. J. Chen, *"Effects of Lactobacillus kefiranofaciens M1 Isolated from Kefir Grains on Germ-Free Mice,"* PLoS One 8, no. 11 (November 11, 2013): e78789, www.ncbi.nlm.nih.gov/pubmed/24244362.

33. Tetsu Sugimura, Kenta Jounai, Konomi Ohshio, Takaaki Tanaka, Masahiro Suwa, and Daisuke Fujiwara, "Immunomodulatory Effect of *Lactococcus lactis JCM5805* on Human Plasmacytoid Dendritic Cells," *Clinical Immunology* 149, no. 3 (December 2013): 509–518, www.ncbi.nlm.nih.gov/pubmed/24239838; M. C. Franco, M. A. Golowczyc, G. L. De Antoni, P. F. Perez, M. Humen, and M. de los Angeles Serradell, "Administration of Kefir-Fermented Milk Protects Mice Against *Giardia intestinalis* Infection," *Journal of Medical Microbiology* 62, pt. 12 (December 2013): 1815–1822, www.ncbi.nlm.nih.gov/pubmed/24072759.

34. H. L. Chen et al., "Kefir Improves Fatty Liver Syndrome by Inhibiting the Lipogenesis Pathway in Leptin-Deficient ob/ob Knockout Mice," *International Journal of Obesity* (London) (December 16, 2013), www.ncbi.nlm.nih.gov/pubmed/24335764.

35. M. Ghoneum and J. Gimzewski, "Apoptotic Effect of a Novel Kefir Product, PFT, on Multidrug-Resistant Myeloid Leukemia Cells via a Hole-Piercing Mechanism," *International Journal of Oncology* 44, no. 3 (March 2014): 830–837, www.ncbi.nlm.nih.gov/pubmed/24430613.

36. G. R. Punaro et al., "Kefir Administration Reduced Progression of Renal Injury in STZ-Diabetic Rats by Lowering Oxidative Stress," *Nitric Oxide* 37 (January 6, 2014): 53–60, www.ncbi.nlm.nih.gov/pubmed/24406684.

37. H. Watanabe, N. Kashimot, J. Kajimura, and K. Kamiya, "A Miso (Japanese soybean paste) Diet Conferred Greater Protection Against Hypertension Than a Sodium Chloride Diet in Dahl Salt-Sensitive Rats," *Hypertension Research* 29, no. 9 (September 2006): 731–738, www.ncbi.nlm.nih.gov/pubmed/17249529.

38. Hiromitsu Watanabe, "Beneficial Biological Effects of Miso with Reference to Radiation Injury, Cancer, and Hypertension," *Journal of Toxicologic Pathology* 26, no. 2 (June 2013): 91–103, www.ncbi.nlm.nih.gov/pubmed/23914051.

39. K. Shiraki, K. Une, R. Yano, S. Otani, A. Mimeoka, and H. Watanabe, "Inhibition by Long-Term Fermented Miso of Induction of Pulmonary Adenocarcinoma by Diisopropanolnitrosamine in Wistar Rats," *Hiroshima Journal*

of Medical Science 52, no. 1 (March 2003): 9–13, www.ncbi.nlm.nih.gov/pubmed/12701648.

40. A. Ito, H. Watanabe, and N. Basaran, "Effects of Soy Products in Reducing Risk of Spontaneous and Neutron-Induced Liver Tumors in Mice," *International Journal of Oncology* 2, no. 5 (May 1993): 773–776.

41. Seiichiro Yamamoto et al., "Frequent Miso Soup and Isoflavone Consumption Is Associated with a Reduced Risk of Breast Cancer in Japanese Women," *Journal of the National Cancer Institute* 95, no. 12 (June 18, 2003): 906–913, www.greenmedinfo.com/article/frequent-miso-soup-and-isoflavone-consumption-associated-reduced-risk-breast; Sayer Ji, "The Amazing Healing Properties of Fermented Foods," GreenMedInfo, April 6, 2012, www.greenmedinfo.com/blog/amazing-healing-properties-fermented-foods; T. Gotoh, K. Yamada, A. Ito, H. Yin, T. Kataoka, and K. Dohi, "Chemoprevention of N-Nitroso-N-Methylurea-Induced Rat Mammary Cancer by Miso and Tamoxifen, Alone and in Combination," *Japanese Journal of Cancer Research* 89, no. 5 (May 1998): 487–495, www.ncbi.nlm.nih.gov/pubmed/9685851; Watanabe, "Beneficial Biological Effects of Miso with Reference to Radiation Injury, Cancer, and Hypertension"; Margie King, "Miso Protects Against Radiation, Cancer, and Hypertension," GreenMedInfo, August 20, 2013, www.greenmedinfo.com/blog/miso-protects-against-radiation-cancer-and-hypertension.

42. M. Tolonen, M. Taipale, B. Viander, J. M Pihlava, H. Kornonen, and E. L. Ryhänen, "Plant-Derived Biomolecules in Fermented Cabbage," *Journal of Agricultural Chemistry* 50, no. 23 (November 6, 2002): 6798–6803, www.ncbi.nlm.nih.gov/pubmed/12405778.

43. Alison Evert, "Phytochemicals," MedlinePlus, May 5, 2011, www.nlm.nih.gov/medlineplus/ency/imagepages/19303.htm.

44. F. Breidt Jr. and J. M. Caldwell, "Survival of *Escheria coli* O157:H7 in Cucumber Fermentation Brines," *Journal of Food Science* 76, no. 3 (April 2011): 198–203, www.ncbi.nlm.nih.gov/pubmed/21535844.

45. "Shigellosis," Centers for Disease Control and Prevention, www.cdc.gov/nczved/divisions/dfbmd/diseases/shigellosis.

46. H. Chon and B. Choi, "The Effects of a Vegetable-Derived Probiotic Lactic Acid Bacterium on the Immune Response," *Microbiology and Immunology* 54, no. 4 (April 2010): 228–236, www.ncbi.nlm.nih.gov/pubmed/20377751.

47. V. K. Bajpai, S. C. Kang, and K. H. Baek, "Microbial Fermentation of Cabbage by a Bacterial Strain of *Pectobacterium atrosepticum* for the Production of Bioactive Material Against Candida Species," *Journal de Mycologie Medicale* 22, no. 1 (March 2012): 21–29, www.ncbi.nlm.nih.gov/pubmed/23177810.

48. A. W. Nichols, "Probiotics and Athletic Performance: A Systematic Review," *Current Sports Medicine Reports* 6, no. 4 (July 2007): 269–273, www.ncbi.nlm.nih.gov/pubmed/17618005.

49. Dawei Gao, Zhengrong Gao, and Guanghua Zhu, "Antioxidant Effects of *Lactobacillus plantarum* via Activation of Transcription Factor Nrf2," *Food and Function* 4, no. 6 (June 4, 2013): 982, www.ncbi.nlm.nih.gov/pubmed /23681127.

50. Y. H. Ju et al., "Estrogenic Effects of Extracts from Cabbage, Fermented Cabbage, and Acidified Brussels Sprouts on Growth and Gene Expression of Estrogen-Dependent Human Breast Cancer (MCF-7) Cells," *Journal of Agricultural Food Chemistry* 48, no. 10 (October 2000): 4628–4634, www.ncbi .nlm.nih.gov/pubmed/11042710.

51. "Sauerkraut," German Food Guide, www.germanfoodguide.com /sauerkraut.cfm.

52. H. C. Mei et al., "Immunomodulatory Activity of *Lactococcus lactis A17* from Taiwan Fermented Cabbage in OVA-Sensitized BALB/c Mice," *Evidence-Based Complementary and Alternative Medicine* 2013, no. 8 (March 7, 2013): 1–11, www.ncbi.nlm.nih.gov/pubmed/23401710.

53. J. Ge et al., "Paracin 1.7, a Bacteriocin Produced by *Lactobacillus paracasei HD1.7* Isolated from Chinese Cabbage Sauerkraut, a Traditional Chinese Fermented Vegetable Food," *Wei Sheng Wu Xue Bao* 49, no. 5 (May 2009): 609–616, www.ncbi.nlm.nih.gov/pubmed/19637568.

54. C. Y. Wang, P. R. Lin, C. C. Ng, and Y. T. Shyu, "Probiotic Properties of *Lactobacillus* Strains Isolated from the Feces of Breast-Fed Infants and Taiwanese Pickled Cabbage," *Anaerobe* 16, no. 6 (December 2010): 578–585, www .ncbi.nlm.nih.gov/pubmed/20951815.

55. Z. Yu, X. Zhang, S. Li, C. Li, D. Li, and Z. Yang, "Evaluation of Probiotic Properties of *Lactobacillus plantarum* Strains Isolated from Chinese Sauerkraut," *World Journal of Microbiology and Biotechnology* 29, no. 3 (March 2013): 489–498, www.ncbi.nlm.nih.gov/pubmed/223117677.

56. Ross Grant, "Fermenting Sauerkraut Foments a Cancer Fighter," *Health Scout New Reporter*, October 24, 2002, www.lifeclinic.com/ams/healthnews/ article_view.asp?story=509840.

57. Sandor Ellix Katz, *Wild Fermentation: The Flavor, Nutrition, and Craft of Live-Culture Foods* (White River Junction, VT: Chelsea Green, 2003), 50.

58. Jinhee Cho, Dongyun Lee, Changnam Yang, Jonhin Jeon, Jeongho Kim, and Hongui Han, "Microbial Population Dynamics of Kimchi, a Fermented Cabbage Product," *FEMS Microbiology Letters* 257, no. 2 (April 2006): 262–267, www.ncbi.nlm.nih.gov/pubmed/16553862.

59. Kun-Young Park, Ji-Kang Jeong, Yong-Eun Lee, and James W. Daily, "Health Benefits of Kimchi (Korean fermented vegetables) as a Probiotic Food," *Journal of Medicinal Food* 17, no. 1 (January 2014): 6–20, www.ncbi.nlmn.ih.gov/pubmed/24456350.

60. M. K. Park et al., "*Lactobacillus plantarum DK119* as a Probiotic Confers Protection Against Influenza Virus by Modulating Innate Immunity," *PLos One* 8, no. 10 (October 4, 2013): e75368, www.ncbi.nlm.nih.gov/pubmed/24124485.

61. Ibid.

62. I. H. Jung, M. A. Jung, E. J. Kim, M. J. Han, and D. H. Kim, "*Lactobacillus pentosus var. plantarum C29* Protects Scopolamine-Induced Memory Deficit in Mice," *Journal of Applied Microbiology* 113, no. 6 (December 2012): 1498–1506, www.ncbi.nlm.nih.gov/pubmed/22925033.

63. T. J. Won et al., "Oral Administration of *Lactobacillus* Strains from Kimchi Inhibits Atopic Dermatitis in NC/Nga Mice," *Journal of Applied Microbiology* 110, no. 5 (May 2011): 1195–1202, www.ncbi.nlm.nih.gov/pubmed/21338447.

64. "Kombucha Culture Instructions," Sproutmaster, www.sproutmaster.com/Article-Kombucha.pdf.

65. I. Vina, P. Semjonovs, R. Linde, and I. Denina, "Current Evidence on Physiological Activity and Expected Health Effects of Kombucha Fermented Beverage," *Journal of Medicinal Food* 17, no. 2 (February 2014): 179–188, www.ncbi.nlm.nih.gov/pubmed/24192111.

66. S. Bhattacharya, R. Gachhui, and P. C. Sil, "Effect of Kombucha, a Fermented Black Tea in Attenuating Oxidative Stress Mediated Tissue Damage in Alloxan Induced Diabetic Rats," *Food and Chemical Toxicology* 60 (October 2013): 328–340, www.ncbi.nlm.nih.gov/pubmed/23907022.

67. Fardin Barati et al., "Histopathological and Clinical Evaluation of Kombucha Tea and Nitrofurazone on Cutaneous Full-Thickness Wounds Healing in Rats: An Experimental Study," *Diagnostic Pathology* 8, no. 1 (July 17, 2013): 120, www.ncbi.nlm.nih.gov/pubmed/23866960.

Appendix: The Cutting-Edge Research

1. S. Hempel et al., "Probiotics for the Prevention and Treatment of Antibiotic-Associated Diarrhea: A Systematic Review and Meta-Analysis," *Journal of the American Medical Association* 307, no. 18 (May 9, 2012): 1959–1969, www.ncbi.nlm.nih.gov/pubmed/22571464.

2. G. Ayala, W. I. Escobedo-Hinojosa, C. F. de la Cruz-Herrera, and I. Romero, "Exploring Alternative Treatments for *Helicobacter pylori* Infection," *World Journal of Gastroenterology* 20, no. 6 (February 14, 2014): 1450–1469, www.ncbi.nlm.nih.gov/pubmed/24587621.

3. E. Lonnermark et al., "Intake of *Lactobacillus plantarum* Reduces Certain Gastrointestinal Symptoms During Treatment with Antibiotics," *Journal of Clinical Gastroenterology*, February 2010, http://www.ncbi.nlm.nih.gov/pubmed /19727002.

4. M. Shu et al., "Fermentation of Propionibacterium Acnes, a Commensal Bacterium in the Human Skin Microbiome, as Skin Probiotics Against Methicillin-Resistant *Staphylococcus aureus*." *PLoS One* 2013, http://www .ncbi.nlm.nih.gov/pubmed/23405142.

5. Ananya Mandal, "What Are Cytokines?" *NewsMedical*, May 17, 2014, www.news-medical.net/health/What-are-Cytokines.aspx.

6. Logan, *The Brain Diet*, 114.

7. G. S. Jensen et al., "A Double-Blind Placebo-Controlled Randomized Pilot Study: A Consumption of a High-Metabolite Immunogen from Yeast Culture Has Beneficial Effects on Erythrocyte Health and Mucosal Immune Protection in Healthy Subjects," *Open Nutritional Journal* 2 (2008): 68–75.

8. Nina Lincoff, "Gut Bacteria May Cause Inflammation in Rheumatoid Arthritis," HealthlineNews, November 8, 2013, www.healthline.com/health -news/arthritis-gut-bacteria-may-trigger-ra-110813.

9. Logan, *The Brain Diet*, 115.

10. P. Hlivak et al., "One Year Application of Probiotic Strain *Enterococcus faecium M-74* Decreases in Serum Cholesterol Levels," *Bratislavske Lekarske Listy*, 2005, www.ncbi.nlm.nih.gov/pubmed/16026136.

11. M. L. Jones, "Cholesterol Lowering and Inhibition of Sterol Absorption by *Lactobacillus reuteri NCIMB 30242*: A Randomized Controlled Trial," *European Journal of Clinical Nutrition*, November 2012, www.ncbi.nlm.nih .gov/22990854.

12. A. J. Nauta et al., "Relevance of Pre- and Postnatal Nutrition to Development and Interplay Between the Microbiota and Metabolic and Immune Systems," *American Journal of Clinical Nutrition*, August 2013, www.ncbi.nlm .nih.gov/pubmed/23824726.

13. T. Poutahidis et al., "Probiotic Microbes Sustain Youthful Serum Testosterone Levels and Testicular Size in Aging Mice," *PLoS One*, January 2, 2014, www.ncbi.nlm.nih.gov/pubmed/24392159.

14. "Yogurt," Wikipedia, http://en.wikipedia.org/wiki/Yogurt.

15. L. Varga, J. Süle, and P. Nagy, "Short Communication: Survival of the Characteristic Microbiota in Probiotic Fermented Camel, Cow, Goat, and

Sheep Milks During Refrigerated Storage," *Journal of Dairy Science* 97, no. 4 (April 2014): 2039–2044.

16. Y. Kim et al., "Fermentation of Soy Milk via *Lactobacillus plantarum* Improves Dysregulated Lipid Metabolism in Rats on a High Cholesterol Diet," *PLos One* 9, no. 2 (February 10, 2014): e88231, www.ncbi.nlm.nih.gov /pubmed/24520358.

17. M. Kobayashi, R. Hirahata, S. Egusa, and M. Fukuda, "Hypocholesterolemic Effects of Lactic Acid-Fermented Soymilk on Rats Fed a High Cholesterol Diet," *Nutrients* 4, no. 9 (September 2012): 1304–1316, www.ncbi.nlm.nih.gov /pubmed/23112918.

18. Cristina Martínez-Villaluenga et al., "Multifunctional Properties of Soy Milk Fermented by *Enterococcus faecium* Strains Isolated from Raw Soy Milk," *Journal of Agricultural Food Chemistry* 60, no. 41 (October 17, 2012): 10235–10244, www.ncbi.nlm.nih.gov/pubmed/22978423.

19. S. S. Chiang and T. M. Pan, "Antiosteoporotic Effects of *Lactobacillus*-Fermented Soy Skim Milk on Bone Mineral Density and the Microstructure of Femoral Bone in Ovariectomized Mice," *Journal of Agricultural Food Chemistry* 59, no. 14 (July 27, 2011): 7734–7742, www.ncbi.nlm.nih.gov/pubmed /21668014.

20. Cox, *The Essential Book of Fermentation*, 22.

21. H. Maeda, Zhu, Omura, Suzuki, and Kitamura, "Effects of an Exopolysaccharide (kefiran) on Lipids, Blood Pressure, Blood Glucose, and Constipation."

22. H. L. Chen et al., "Kefir Improves Fatty Liver Syndrome by Inhibiting the Lipogenesis Pathway in Leptin-Deficient ob/ob Knockout Mice."

23. A. Ito, Watanabe, and Basaran, "Effects of Soy Products in Reducing Risk of Spontaneous and Neutron-Induced Liver Tumors in Mice."

24. Yamamoto et al., "Frequent Miso Soup and Isoflavone Consumption Is Associated with a Reduced Risk of Breast Cancer in Japanese Women"; Ji, "The Amazing Healing Properties of Fermented Foods."

25. T. Gotoh, Yamada, Ito, Yin, Kataoka, and Dohi, "Chemoprevention of N-Nitroso-N-Methylurea-Induced Rat Mammary Cancer by Miso and Tamoxifen, Alone and in Combination."

26. Ibid.

27. Watanabe, "Beneficial Biological Effects of Miso with Reference to Radiation Injury, Cancer, and Hypertension."

28. King, "Miso Protects Against Radiation, Cancer, and Hypertension."

29. Tolonen, Taipale, Viander, Pihlava, Korhonen, and Ryhanen, "Plant-Derived Biomolecules in Fermented Cabbage."

30. Grant, "Fermenting Sauerkraut Foments a Cancer Fighter."

31. Ibid.

32. Won et al., "Oral Administration of *Lactobacillus* Strains from Kimchi Inhibits Atopic Dermatitis in NC/Nga Mice."

33. S. M. Lee, "Effects of Kimchi Supplementation on Blood Pressure and Cardiac Hypertrophy with Varying Sodium Content in Spontaneously Hypertensive Rats," *Nutrition in Research and Practice* 6, no. 4 (August 2012): 315–321, www.ncbi.nlm.nih.gov/pubmed/22977685.

34. F. Barati et al., "Histopathological and Clinical Evaluation of Kombucha Tea and Nitrofurazone on Cutaneous Full-Thickness Wounds Healing in Rats: An Experimental Study," *Diagnostic Pathology* 8, no. 1 (July 17, 2013): 120, www.ncbi.nlm.nih.gov/pubmed/23866960.

35. N. F. Fu et al., "Clearance of Free Silica in Rat Lungs by Spraying with Chinese Herbal Kombucha," *Evidence-Based Complementary and Alternative Medicine* 2013, no. 7 (2013): 1–9, www.ncbi.nlm.nih.gov/pubmed/24023583.

36. Y. Wang et al., "Hepatoprotective Effects of Kombucha Tea: Identification of Functional Strains and Quantification of Functional Components," *Journal of the Science of Food and Agriculture* 94, no. 2 (January 30, 2014): 265–272, www.ncbi.nlm.nih.gov/pubmed/23716136.

37. Alan J. Marsh, Orla O'Sullivan, Colin Hill, R. Paul Ross, and Paul D. Cotter, "Sequence-Based Analysis of the Bacterial and Fungal Compositions of Multiple Kombucha (tea fungus) Samples," *Food Microbiology* 38, no. 4 (April 2014): 171–178, www.ncbi.nlm.nih.gov/pubmed/24290641.

About the Author

Michelle Schoffro Cook, PhD, DNM, DHS, ROHP, is the author of seventeen health books, including the international bestsellers *60 Seconds to Slim*, *The Ultimate pH Solution*, and *The 4-Week Ultimate Body Detox Plan*. She holds advanced degrees in natural health, holistic and orthomolecular nutrition, and traditional natural medicine, and has twenty-five years of experience in the field. Dr. Cook is a board-certified doctor of natural medicine. She received the doctor of humanitarian services designation from the World Organization of Natural Medicine and a World-Leading Intellectual Award for her contribution to natural medicine. She is the publisher of the popular health e-zine *World's Healthiest News* and is a regular blogger for TheProbioticPromise.com, PureFoodWarrior.com, HealthySurvivalist.com, and Care2.com. Check out her websites: DrMichelleCook.com and WorldsHealthiestDiet.com. Subscribe to her free e-zine at WorldsHealthiestDiet.com.

Acknowledgments

Thank you to my wonderful agent and friend, Claire. You're a true visionary and excellent agent. Thanks for all you do to share my books with readers.

Thank you to Renee for your belief in this book and your many editing talents.

Thanks to Kevin Mehring for your excellent title suggestion.

Thanks to the team at Da Capo for all your efforts on design, editing, marketing, promotions, and project management to make *The Probiotic Promise* what it is and will become.

Thanks to my parents, Michael and Deborah Schoffro, for your ongoing belief in me throughout my lifetime.

Thanks, last but definitely not least, to Curtis, my amazing husband and love of my life. I can never thank you for all you do for me and for always treating me like a queen.

Thanks to everyone else who played a role in this book.

Index

Acetaminophen, 240
Acetobacter, 146
Acid bath, 32
Acne, 50
Activia, 136, 137–138
Adenosine triphosphate (ATP),
    185–186
Adrenal exhaustion, 48, 49
Age factor, 125
Aging
    cancer and, 90
    inflammation and, 34, 35,
        155–156
    of men, 233
    probiotics for, 101–102, 155–156,
        233
    skin, 155–156
    vitamins for, 102
AIDS, 72, 73–74
Alcohol
    Candida from, 27
    fermentation by, 145
Allergic rhinoconjunctivitis (ARC),
    84
Allergies
    Candida from, 30
    case study on, 79–80
    natural remedies for, 80
    probiotic fillers and, 125
    probiotics for, 80, 84–85, 116, 231
    See also Food sensitivity

Almonds
    Almond Ricotta Cheese, 200–201
    cream from, 217–218
    yogurt from, 186–192
Aloe vera, 45
Alpha lipoic acid, 102, 140
Alzheimer's disease, 36, 88–90
Ampicillin, 57
Amylase, 43
Animal products. See Dairy products;
    Meat
Anise carrots, 211–212
Antacids, 28
Antibacterial products, 48, 50
Antibiotics
    Candida from, 28
    diarrhea from, 60–63, 132 (table),
        229
    probiotic dosage with, 129–130
    probiotics versus, 13–14, 58–60
    skin problems and, 50, 230
    superbug creation and, 54–57
    superbug resistance to, 49–54
    veterinary, 51
Antioxidants, 89, 101–102
Anxiety, 85–86, 132 (table), 231
Apples
    apple cider vinegar, 43
    Apple-Cabbage Kraut, 171,
        210–211
    benefits of, 40–41

ARC. *See* Allergic rhinoconjunctivitis
Arthritis, 87–88, 232, 234
Artificial sweeteners, 185
Asthma, 36
Athletic performance, 168, 186
ATP. *See* Adenosine triphosphate
Autoimmune disorders, 25, 33, 182

Bacillus subtilis, 76
Bacteria
    benefits of, 18
    count in body, 17
    good, bad and "swing voter,"
        19–20
    HMP for, 20–22
    superbugs, 49–57, 76
Bacterial overgrowth
    process of, 33
    symptoms of, 25–26
    testing for, 24
    See also Gut health
Bacteriocin, 65, 68, 169
Bacteriophages, 53
Bacteroides, 34, 116, 117
Basil–Pumpkin Seed Soft Cheese,
    203–204
Bassler, Bonnie L., 47, 79
BDNF. *See* Brain-derived
    neurotrophic factor
Beer, 27
Belaiche, Paul, 77
Beverages
    alcohol intake, 27
    coconut milk, 195
    green tea kombucha, 195–198
    herbal tea, 43, 119
    smoothies, 193–194
    water intake, 44, 108, 130
Bifidobacteria, 115–118

Bifidobacteria bifiform,
    B. bifiform, 64
Bifidobacterium animalis,
    B. animalis, 68, 101, 137
Bifidobacterium bifidum,
    B. bifidum, 68, 116
Bifidobacterium bifidus,
    B. bifidus, 43
Bifidobacterium breve,
    B. breve, 92, 97, 116–117
Bifidobacterium infantis,
    B. infantis, 97–98, 117
Bifidobacterium lactis, B. lactis
    about, 117–118
    for heart disease, 100
    for IBS, 97–98
    for pregnancy, 101
    in yogurt, 138
Bifidobacterium longum,
    B. longum, 86, 92, 97, 118
Bifidus Regularis, B. L. Regularis,
    136–137
Bile, 32–33
Biofilm, 68
BioFrontiers Institute, 22
Birth control, 28
Bjeldanes, Leonard, 238
Black and Blue Berry Gelato,
    220–221
Bloating, 20, 36, 95, 141
Blood
    leaky gut viral access to, 36
    nutrient absorption in, 32
    poisoning, 113
    white blood cells, 74, 111
Blood pressure, 164, 239
Blood sugar imbalance, 28, 103, 104,
    148
    See also Diabetes

Blueberries, 193, 220–221
Boulard, Henri, 119
Bowel movements
    constipation, 26, 44–46, 96
    importance of, 41, 44
    stool testing, 24
    See also Colon; Diarrhea
Brain disease
    fermented foods for, 150, 174
    leaky gut and, 36
    probiotics for, 88–90, 232
Brain-derived neurotrophic factor
    (BDNF), 231
Brands
    probiotic, 126–128, 129
    yogurt, 135–138
Bread, sourdough, 147
Breast cancer
    constipation and, 26
    miso for, 165, 237
    soy myths and, 159
    yogurt for, 149
Brining, 144
Budget, 177
Buhner, Stephen Harrod, 52, 54, 103
Bulgaria, 148

Cabbage
    kimchi, 172–175, 214–216,
        238–239
    sauerkraut, 166–172, 208–211,
        238
Caesar salad dressing, 205
Calcium, 32, 115, 155
Campylobacter jejuni, C. jejuni, 116,
    117
Canada
    anxiety research from, 86
    cancer research from, 16, 91

colitis research from, 94
    heart disease research from, 233
    MRSA research from, 67
Cancer
    aging and, 90
    breast, 26, 149, 159, 165, 237
    case studies, 15–17, 139–141
    chemotherapy for, 63, 90–91, 132
        (table)
    colon, 91, 154, 164, 165
    diet for, 16, 140, 237–238
    fermented foods for, 149, 154–155,
        162, 164–165, 168, 237–238
    genetics and, 90
    kefir for, 162
    liver, 165, 237–238
    lung, 164–165, 238
    miso for, 164–165, 237–238
    natural remedies for, 16–17, 140
    probiotics for, 16, 90–91, 112, 149
    prostate, 159
    radiation therapy for, 90–91, 238
    sauerkraut for, 168, 238
    skin, 139–141
    smoking and, 91
    stomach, 15–17
    yogurt benefits for, 149, 154–155
Candida
    causes of, 27–30, 48, 74
    fermented foods for, 74, 167, 176,
        230–231
    natural remedies for, 48–49, 75–78
    probiotics for, 48, 119
    symptoms of, 26–27
Candida albicans, 26, 27
Candidiasis, 26–27
Canning, 170
Carbapenem-resistant *Enterobacteri-
    aceae* (CRE), 55, 57

Carbapenem-resistant *Klebsiella pneumonia* (CRKP), 55
Carrots, 211–212
Case studies
  allergies, 79–80
  chronic fatigue, 47–49
  depression, 103–105
  IBS, 1–3
  skin cancer, 139–141
  stomach cancer, 15–17
Cashew-Thyme Soft Cheese, 202–203
Cashews
  cheese from, 200, 201–202,
    204–205
  cream from, 217–218
  frozen yogurt from, 221–222
  gelato from, 220–221
  ice cream from, 219–220, 223
  yogurt from, 188–192
CD4 count, 74
CDC. *See* Centers for Disease Control
  and Prevention
Celiac disease, 20, 36, 93–94, 96
Cellulase, 43
CENTER. *See* Clinical Enteric
  Neuroscience Translational and
  Epidemiological Research
Centers for Disease Control and
  Prevention (CDC)
  on antibacterial products, 50
  on arthritis, 87
  on heart disease, 99
  on superbugs, 54–55
Cephalexin, 59
CFUs. *See* Colony-forming units
Cheese, 38, 112, 118
  See also Dairy-free cheese
Chemotherapy, 63, 90–91, 132 (table)
Chewing, 31–32, 42

Chickens, 56, 57
Children. *See* Infants and children
Chile, 66, 230
Chilis, 212, 213
China
  fermented foods from, 168–169,
    175
  research from, 59, 240
Chlorinated water, 28, 131
Chocolate smoothie, 193–194
Cholera, 117
Cholesterol
  probiotics for, 100, 112, 132
    (table), 232–233
  soy yogurt and, 154, 235
Chronic fatigue, 25, 47–49
Clinical Enteric Neuroscience Trans-
  lational and Epidemiological
  Research (CENTER) Group, 97
Clostridium difficile, C. diff
  aggressiveness of, 67
  diseases linked to, 94, 113
  probiotics for, 113, 114, 116, 119
Clostridium perfringens, 41
Coconut
  cream, 216–217
  ice cream, 218–219, 222–223
  milk, 195
  oil, 76, 140
Colds, 14, 50, 69, 132 (table)
Colic, 96
Colitis, 36, 94, 118
Colon
  cancer, 91, 154, 164, 165
  cleanses, 46
  colitis, 36, 94, 118
  Crohn's disease, 36, 94
  diverticulosis, 98–99
  IBD, 36, 94

IBS, 1–3, 95–98, 132 (table)
Colony-forming units (CFUs), 120,
    121, 123
Company reputation, 121–122
    See also Brands
Constipation, 26, 44–46, 96
Cosmetics, 155–156
Cramping, 1–3, 36, 95
Cranberry juice, 66, 230
CRE. See Carbapenem-resistant
    Enterobacteriaceae
C-reactive protein (CRP), 93, 101,
    233
Cream, 216–218
Creamsicle Ice Cream, 219–220
Creamy Dairy-Free Yogurt Cheese,
    199
CRKP. See Carbapenem-resistant
    Klebsiella pneumonia
Crohn's disease, 36, 94
CRP. See C-reactive protein
Cultured Anise Carrots, 211–212
Cultured Coconut Cream, 216
Cultured Coconut Milk, 195
Cultured foods. See Fermented foods
Curcumin, 17, 140
Curtis's Chocolate Banana Pro
    Smoothie, 193–194
Cytokines, 82–83, 231

Dairy products
    arthritis from, 234
    cheese, 38, 112, 118
    IBS from, 95
    inflammation from, 37–39
    probiotics to digest, 111, 112
    problems overview, 152–153
    sensitivity to, 80, 125, 182
    superbugs rise in, 51

See also Yogurt
Dairy-free cheese
    Almond Ricotta Cheese, 200–201
    Basil-Pumpkin Seed Soft Cheese,
        203–204
    cashew, 200, 201–202, 204–205
    Cashew-Thyme Soft Cheese,
        202–203
    Roasted Red Pepper Soft Cheese,
        201–202
    yogurt, 199
Dairy-Free Cream, 217–218
Dairy-Free, Probiotic Rich Caesar
        Salad Dressing, 205
Dairy-Free Whey, 188
Dairy-Free Yogurt, 186–188
    about, 151–157, 234–235, 236
    savory Greek-style, 188–191
    sweet, 191–192
Dandelion, 76
Danone, 136–138
David, Lawrence, 38
Dementia, 89, 174
Dental health, 63, 114, 132 (table)
Depression, 85–86, 103–105, 231
Dermatitis, 239
Desserts
    cream, 216–218
    frozen yogurt, 221–222
    gelato, 220–221
    ice cream, 218–220, 222–223
Diabetes
    Candida from, 28
    causes and types, 92
    fatty liver disease and, 237
    fermented foods for, 162–163, 176
    leaky gut syndrome and, 93
    probiotics for, 92–93
Diagnostic tests, 24

Diarrhea
  antibiotic-related, 60–63, 132
    (table), 229
  probiotics for, 60–63, 119, 132
    (table)
  traveler's, 99, 132 (table)
Diet
  for cancer, 16, 140, 237–238
  Candida from, 28, 29
  chronic fatigue from, 48
  for constipation, 44
  depression and, 103–104
  diabetes and, 92
  frozen food in, 2
  heart disease and, 99
  intermediate bacteria and, 19
  magnesium in, 45
  meat in, 37–39
  meat-free protein in, 39–41
  nutrient absorption and, 33
  prebiotics in, 107–109
  SAD, 33, 38, 113
  See also Dairy products;
    Fermented foods; Food
    sensitivity; Sugar
Digestion
  improvement strategies, 42–43,
    236
  process, 31–34
Digestive disorders
  antacids and, 28
  bloating, 20, 36, 95, 141
  celiac disease, 20, 36, 93–94, 96
  colitis, 36, 94, 118
  cramping, 1–3, 36, 95
  diverticulosis, 98–99
  gastritis, 64–66, 67, 230
  Giardia, 162
  hydrochloric acid and, 29

  IBS, 1–3, 95–98, 132 (table)
  in infants and children, 96
  leaky gut syndrome and, 36, 83
  stress and, 42, 83, 85–86
  ulcers, 64–66, 67, 198, 230
Diverticulosis, 98–99
Douches, 72, 131
D-ribose, 185–186
Drugs
  acetaminophen, 240
  ampicillin, 57
  for arthritis, 87
  birth control, 28
  Candida from, 28–29
  cephalexin, 59
  erythromycin, 59
  gentamicin, 59
  kombucha and, 239, 240
  methicillin, 55
  miso and, 237
  nitrofurazone, 176, 239
  NSAIDs, 64
  oxytetracycline, 56, 59
  probiotic contraindications with,
    124
  streptomycin, 56, 57, 59
  sulfanomides, 57
  symptom suppression by, 10
  tamoxifen, 237
  tetracycline, 53, 57, 59
  triclosan, 50
  vancomycin, 59
  for wound treatment, 176, 239
  See also Antibiotics
DuPont Nutrition and Health, 61
Dysbiosis, 33

E. coli
  apples and, 41

probiotics for, 112, 114, 118, 119
sauerkraut for, 166–167, 169
soy for, 156
as suberbug, 55, 57
Ear infections, 70
Echinacea, 174
Eczema, 36, 84
EGCG. *See* Epigallocatechin gallate
Elderberries, 174
Elderly care, 70, 128, 149
    See also Aging
Emotional disorders, 85–86,
    103–105, 231
Emotional processing, 89
England, 97
Enterococcus, 41, 78, 113, 235
Enterococcus faecium, 100, 232–233
Enzymes, 32, 42, 114
Epigallocatechin gallate (EGCG),
    206
Equipment, 183, 207
Erythromycin, 59
Essiac, 16
Estrogen, 30, 149, 158–159, 168

Factory farms, 51
Fatigue, chronic, 25, 47–49
Fatty liver disease, 237
Fermentation
    by alcohol, 145
    by brining, 144
    canning and, 170
    pickling and, 169, 170
    by probiotic powder, 144
    process, 119, 171–172, 238
    by sodium grain or legume paste,
        146–147
    sugar and, 171–172, 185–186
    types of, 143–147

by vinegar, 146
by whey starter, 145
by yogurt starter, 144–145
Fermented foods
    athletic performance and, 168
    benefits of homemade, 177–180
    bifidobacteria family in, 116
    from China, 168–169, 175
    dead or live cultures in, 9,
        133–135, 170, 176, 178
    equipment for, 183, 207
    from Germany, 168–169
    for infants, 150, 233
    ingredients for, 183–186
    from Korea, 172–173
    lactobacilli family in, 111
    origins of, 142–143, 168–169
    from Russia, 148, 175
    from Turkey, 147, 161
Fermented foods, by illness
    for brain disease, 150, 174
    for cancer, 149, 154–155, 162,
        164–165, 168, 237–238
    for Candida, 74, 167, 176,
        230–231
    for diabetes, 162–163, 176
    for fatty liver disease, 237
    for flu, 174, 238
    for food poisoning, 150, 166–167
    for *H. pylori*, 149–150
    for heart disease, 153–154, 168
    for kidney health, 171
    for liver disease, 165, 237–238,
        240
    for metabolic syndrome, 148
    for nutrient absorption, 149, 164
    for osteoporosis, 155
    for respiratory infection, 148–149,
        239–240

Fermented foods, by illness
(continued)
for skin problems, 155–156, 174,
176–177, 239
for wound treatment, 176–177,
239–240
Fermented foods, by type
apple cider vinegar, 43
carrots, 211–212
cheese, 38, 112, 118
cheese, dairy-free, 199–205
coconut cream, 216–217
coconut ice cream, 218–219,
222–223
coconut milk, 195
green bean pickles, 213
hot sauce, 212
kefir, 161–163, 236–237
kimchi, 172–175, 214–216,
238–239
kombucha, 175–177, 239–240
miso, 163–165, 237–238
onions, 214
salad dressings, 205–207
sauerkraut, 166–172, 208–211,
238
sourdough bread, 147
tofu, 165
whey, 145, 186, 188, 190–191
See also Yogurt
Fermented Green Tea (Kombucha),
195–198
Fermented Onions, 214
Fiber
constipation and, 44
diverticulosis and, 98–99
prebiotics and, 107, 108, 109
Fibromyalgia, 87
Finland, 70, 101, 238

Fish, 45
Fish oil, 104
5-HTP, 104
Flu
antibiotics for, 14
fermented foods for, 174, 238
natural remedies for, 174
probiotics for, 132 (table), 238
Food poisoning
fermented foods for, 150, 166–167
probiotics for, 117, 132 (table), 150
Food sensitivity
to dairy, 80, 125, 182
to gluten, 20, 36, 93–94, 96, 182
probiotic fillers and, 125
FOS. See Fructooligosaccharides
Free radicals, 77, 89, 101–102
Frozen food, 2
Frozen yogurt, 221–222
Fructooligosaccharides (FOS), 92,
100, 108–109
Fruit
about, 183–184
antibiotics used on, 56–57
creamsicle, 219–220
freshness preservation of, 141–142,
179
gelato, 220–221
pops, 222
smoothies, 193–194
See also Apples
Fungal infections, 72, 74–78
See also Candida
Fungi, beneficial, 119

Gallbladder, 32–33
GALT. See Gut-associated lymphoid
tissue
Garlic, 77, 213

Gastritis, 64–66, 67, 230
Gastroenteritis, 113
Gastrointestinal (GI) system, 31–34
Gastrointestinal (GI) tract, 31
　See also Gut health
Gelato, 220–221
Genetics
　brain disease and, 89
　cancer and, 90
　Human Genome Project, 21
　jumping genes, 53
Genistein, 158–159
Gentamicin, 59
German sauerkraut, 168–169
Germophobia, 48, 50
GI system. *See* Gastrointestinal
　system
GI tract. *See* Gastrointestinal tract
Giardia, 162
Ginger, 43, 206
Ginseng, 49
Gluconacetobacter, 240
Glucosinolates, 167, 178, 238
Gluten
　probiotic breakdown of, 93–94,
　　111, 112
　sensitivity, 20, 36, 93–94, 96, 182
　sourdough bread, 147
Gonorrhea, 55–56, 77
Gout, 87
Grain fermentation, 146–147
　See also Gluten
Greek-style yogurt, 188–191
Green bean pickles, 213
Green Chili Hot Sauce, 212
Green powder, 184
Green tea, 195–198, 206–207
Greens, 45
Gut health

apples for, 40–41
GI system and, 31–34
good versus bad bacteria and,
　19–20
imbalances, 24–26
inflammation link to, 34–37,
　82–84, 231
nutrient absorption and, 32, 33
probiotic actions on, 23–24,
　59–60, 65, 106–107
probiotic supplement for, 44–45
role of, 22–24
Gut-associated lymphoid tissue
　(GALT), 34–35

Headaches, 36
Heart disease
　fermented foods for, 153–154, 168
　probiotics for, 99–101, 232–233
Helicobacter pylori, H. pylori
　fermented foods for, 149–150
　probiotics for, 64–66, 67, 112, 132
　　(table), 229–230
Hemicellulase, 43
Herbal remedies. *See* Natural
　remedies
Herpes, 71
HIV. *See* Human immunodeficiency
　virus
HMP. *See* Human Microbiome
　Project
Homocysteine, 101, 148
Hormones
　Candida and, 27, 30
　cytokines and, 231
　depression and, 103–104
　diabetes and, 92
　estrogen, 30, 149, 158–159, 168
　metabolic syndrome and, 148

Hormones *(continued)*
  sauerkraut for, 167
  soy myths on, 157–160
  testosterone, 233
  xenoestrogen, 30, 158–159
Hospital-acquired disease, 57, 69, 113
Hot sauce, 212
Human Genome Project, 21
Human immunodeficiency virus
  (HIV), 35, 71–72, 73–74
Human Microbiome Project (HMP),
  20–22
Hungary, 86
Hydrochloric acid, 29, 32
Hypothyroidism, 28

IBD. *See* Inflammatory bowel disease
IBS. *See* Irritable bowel syndrome
Ice cream, 218–220, 222–223
IgA. *See* Immunoglobulin A
Immune system
  allergies and, 231
  anxiety, depression and, 231
  Candida and, 30
  HIV and, 71–72, 73–74
  inflammation and, 23–24, 231
  kefir for, 161–162
  tumors and, 117
Immunoglobulin A (IgA), 231
India, 74
Infants and children
  allergies in, 84, 233
  antibiotic-related diarrhea in,
    62–63
  brand recommendations for, 128
  digestive disorders in, 96
  fermented foods for, 150, 233
  HIV in, 74
  IBS in, 98

probiotics at pregnancy for, 84,
  101, 110, 115–116
probiotics in, 117
respiratory infection in, 70
Inflammation
  aging and, 34, 35, 155–156
  allergies and, 84–85
  anxiety, depression and, 86, 231
  arthritis and, 87–88, 232, 234
  brain disease and, 232
  colitis and, 94, 118
  cytokines role in, 82–83, 231
  from dairy, 37–39
  depression and, 86
  diabetes and, 93
  diverticulosis and, 98
  gut health link to, 34–37, 82–84,
    231
  health problems from, 81–84
  heart disease and, 82, 100–101,
    233
  HIV and, 35
  immune system and, 23–24
  from meat, 37–39
  probiotic action for, 23–24
  process, 82–83
Inflammatory bowel disease (IBD),
  36, 94
Ingredients, 183–186
Interferons, 112
Intermediate "swing voter" bacteria,
  19–20
Intestinal health. *See* Gut health
Intestinal villi, 32, 33, 83, 93–94
Inulin, 100, 108
Iran, 72, 176, 239
Irritable bowel syndrome (IBS), 1–3,
  95–98, 132 (table)
Isoflavones, 149, 158–160

Isothiocyanates, 167, 178, 238
Italy, 71, 94, 98

Japan
    allergy research in, 85
    cancer research in, 91, 237–238
    kefir research in, 236
    soy yogurt research in, 153–154,
        235
Jensen, Bernard, 20
Ju, Yeong, 172
Jumping genes, 53

Kantvik Active Nutrition, 61
Katz, Sandor Ellix, 139, 173
Kefir, 161–163, 236–237
Kefiran, 236
Keim, Brandon, 51
Kidney health
    adrenal exhaustion, 48, 49
    fermented food for, 171
Kimchi
    benefits of, 173–175, 238–239
    history of, 172–173
    recipe, 214–216
Klebsiella, 55
Kombucha
    benefits of, 175–177, 239–240
    recipe, 195–198
Korea
    fermented foods from, 172–173
    research from, 77, 155–156, 157,
        239

Labels
    accuracy of, 122, 126–128
    live cultures on, 9, 133–135, 170,
        176, 178
    marketing gimmicks on, 136–138

Lactase, 43
Lactic acid, 111, 133, 171–172
Lactobacilli family, 110–115
Lactobacillus acidophilus,
        L. acidophilus, 132 (table)
    about, 111–112
    antibiotics and, 59, 61
    brands, 127
    for diabetes, 92
    for heart disease, 100
    for IBS, 97, 98
    for *S. Aureus*, 68
    in yogurt, 133, 155, 160
Lactobacillus brevis, *L. brevis*, 71,
        112
Lactobacillus bulgaricus,
        L. bulgaricus, 92, 97, 112
Lactobacillus casei, *L. casei*, 132
        (table)
    about, 112
    for allergies, 85
    antibiotics and, 59, 61, 62
    for cancer, 149
    for celiac disease, 94
    for diabetes, 92
    for diverticular disease, 99
    for respiratory infection, 70, 148
Lactobacillus casei Shirota,
        L. casei Shirota, 91, 101
Lactobacillus delbrueckii bulgaricus,
        L. delbrueckii bulgaricus, 59,
        62, 234
Lactobacillus fermentum,
        L. fermentum, 75
Lactobacillus gasseri, *L. gasseri*,
        113
Lactobacillus GG, 62, 101
Lactobacillus helveticus,
        L. helveticus, 86

Lactobacillus johnsonii, L. johnsonii,
  67, 101
Lactobacillus kefiranofaciens,
    L. kefiranofaciens, 236
Lactobacillus kefiri, L. kefiri, 162
Lactobacillus lactis, L. lactis, 68, 101
Lactobacillus mesenteroides,
    L. mesenteroides, 166
Lactobacillus paracasei, L. paracasei,
  132 (table)
  about, 113
  antibiotics and, 59
  for colds, 69
  H. pylori and, 67
  for IBS, 97
  in sauerkraut, 169
  in yogurt, 150, 236
Lactobacillus pentosus var.
  plantarum, 239
Lactobacillus plantarum,
    L. plantarum, 132 (table)
  about, 113–114
  antibiotics and, 59, 62, 229
  for brain disease, 89
  for colds, 69
  for flu, 174, 238
  for food poisoning, 166–167
  for heart disease, 100
  for herpes, 71
  for IBS, 97
  in kimchi, 151, 238
  for metabolic syndrome, 148
  in plant foods, 113–114
  for *S. aureus,* 68
  in yogurt, 154, 160, 236
Lactobacillus reuteri, L. reuteri
  about, 114
  adult effectiveness of, 62, 63
  for arthritis, 87–88

for dental health, 63
for *H. pylori,* 67, 114
for heart disease, 100
for IBS, 98
for male aging, 233
for MRSA, 68
Lactobacillus rhamnosus,
    L. rhamnosus, 132 (table)
  about, 114
  for arthritis, 87–88
  for diabetes, 92
  H. pylori and, 125, 230
  for HIV, 72
  for IBS, 97
  for MRSA, 68
  for pregnancy, 101
  for yeast infections, 75
Lactobacillus salivarius,
    L. salivarius, 16, 111, 115,
    132 (table)
Latvia, 175
Leafy greens, 45
Leaky gut syndrome, 34–35, 36, 83,
  93
Lee, B., 77
Lee, O., 77
Legumes
  fermentation using, 146–147
  as magnesium source, 45
  as protein source, 39
Leuconostoc, 173
Levy Lab, 56
Levy, Stuart, 56
Licorice root, 45, 49
Lifestyle
  brain disease and, 89
  cancer and, 90
  diabetes and, 92
  heart disease and, 99

Lime vinaigrette/marinade,
206–207
Lipase, 43
Listeria, 113, 169
Littman, Dan, 232
Live cultures designation, 9, 133–135,
170, 176, 178
Liver
acetaminophen damage to, 240
cancer, 165, 237–238
digestion process of, 32–33
fatty liver disease, 237
fermented foods for, 165, 237–238,
240
Lou Gehrig's disease, 88–90
Lung cancer, 164–165, 238
See also Respiratory infections
Lupus, 87

Magnesium, 45
Malaysia, 155
Maltose, 27
Mango Frozen Yogurt Pops, 222
Margulis, Lynn, 15
Marinade, 206–207
MCTs. See Medium-chain
triglycerides
Measurements, 225–227
Meat
chicken, 56, 57
inflammation from, 37–39
protein alternatives to, 39–41
superbugs in, 51, 56, 57
Mechnikov, Ilya Ilyich, 148, 236
Medium-chain triglycerides (MCTs),
195, 216, 218
Men
aging of, 233
liver tumors in, 237

prostate cancer in, 159
soy myths and, 159, 160
Meningitis, 77, 113
Menopause, 149, 158
Mercury, 29
Metabolic syndrome, 148
Methicillin-resistant *Staphylococcus
aureus* (MRSA)
locations of, 57
probiotics for, 66–69, 113
proliferation of, 51, 55
Metric conversions, 225–227
Microbial balance, 7, 41
See also Gut health
Microbiome, 21
Mild Cheese, 204–205
Milk, coconut, 195
Minerals
for aging, 102
calcium, 32, 115, 155
for constipation, 45
definition of, 31
magnesium, 45
for osteoporosis, 115, 155
selenium, 102
Mint tea, 43
Miso, 163–165, 237–238
Monosodium glutamate (MSG), 40,
104
MRSA. See Methicillin-resistant
Staphylococcus aureus
MSG. See Monosodium glutamate

Nasal congestion, 79–80, 85
Natural remedies
for allergies, 80
aloe vera, 45
alpha lipoic acid, 102, 140
for cancer, 16–17, 140

Natural remedies *(continued)*
  for Candida, 48–49, 75–78
  coconut oil, 76, 140
  for constipation, 45
  cranberry juice, 66, 230
  curcumin, 17, 140
  dandelion, 76
  for depression, 104
  echinacea, 174
  elderberries, 174
  Essiac, 16
  fish oil, 104
  for flu, 174
  for fungal infections, 75–78
  garlic, 77
  for gastritis, 66, 230
  ginseng, 49
  licorice root, 45, 49
  nettles, 80
  olive leaf, 77
  oregano oil, 77–78
  pokeroot, 140
  resveratrol, 140
  St. John's Wort, 104
  tea, 43
  for ulcers, 66, 230
  for viruses, 75–78
  for yeast infections, 75–78
  yoga, 46
Nausea, 16, 162
Neill, Margeurite, 57
Neisseria, 77
Netherlands, 93
Nettles, 80
New Zealand, 69
Nitrofurazone, 176, 239
Nonsteroidal anti-inflammatory
  drugs (NSAIDs), 64
Nutrient absorption, 32, 33, 149, 164

Nuts
  about, 40, 45, 184
  cheese from, 200–205
  cream from, 217–218
  frozen yogurt from, 221–222
  gelato from, 220–221
  ice cream from, 219–220, 223
  yogurt from, 186–192

Obesity, 159, 237
Oligosaccharides, 108–109, 156–157
Olive leaf, 77
Omega 3 fatty acids, 86, 202, 203
Onions, 214
Orange creamsicle, 219–220
Oregano oil, 77–78
Osteoporosis, 115, 155, 236
Oven temperature, 227
Oxytetracycline, 56, 59

Panush, Richard, 234
Pasteurization, 170, 172, 176, 178
Peppermint tea, 43
Periodontitis, 63, 114, 132 (table)
Peristalsis, 236
Pet products, 128
Phytic acid, 160, 164
Phytonutrients, 149
Pickling
  Garlic Chili Green Bean Pickles,
    213
  process, 169, 170
Plant foods
  L. plantarum in, 113–114
  prebiotics in, 107, 109
  protein in, 39–41, 193
  See also Fruit; Vegetables
Plasmids, 53
Plastic toxins, 30, 159, 183

Pneumococcus, 77
Pokeroot, 140
Poland, 172
Pollan, Michael, 22
Potency, 123, 178
Powders, probiotic, 144
Prebiotics, 107–109, 156–157
Pregnancy
    constipation from, 44
    diabetes from, 92
    probiotics during, 84, 101, 110,
        115–116, 124
Prevotella copri, P. copri, 88, 232
Proanthocyanidins, 193
Probiotic family
    Bifidobacteria, 115–118
    Lactobacilli, 110–115
    Saccharomyces, 119
    Streptococcus, 118–119
Probiotic Jar, 207
Probiotic products, by illness, 132
        (table)
    for aging, 101–102, 155–156, 233
    for AIDS, 72, 73–74
    for allergies, 80, 84–85, 116, 231
    for antibiotic-related diarrhea,
        60–63, 229
    for anxiety, 85–86, 132 (table),
        231
    for arthritis, 87–88, 232
    for brain disease, 88–90, 232
    for *C. diff*, 113, 114, 116, 119
    for cancer, 16, 90–91, 112, 149
    for Candida, 48, 119
    for celiac disease, 93–94
    for chemotherapy, 63, 90–91, 132
        (table)
    for cholesterol, 100, 112, 132
        (table), 232–233

for chronic fatigue, 48
for colds, 14, 50, 69, 132 (table)
for colitis, 94, 118
for constipation, 44–45
for dairy sensitivity, 111, 112
for dental disorders, 63, 114, 132
    (table)
for depression, 85–86, 231
for diabetes, 92–93
for diarrhea, 60–63, 110, 132
    (table)
for diverticulosis, 99
for *E. coli*, 112, 114, 118, 119
for ear infections, 70
for flu, 132 (table), 238
for food poisoning, 117, 132
    (table), 150
for fungal infections, 72, 75–78
for gastritis, 64–66, 67, 230
for gluten breakdown, 93–94, 111,
    112
for gonorrhea, 55–56
for *H. pylori*, 64–66, 67, 112, 132
    (table), 229–230
for heart disease, 99–101, 232–233
for herpes, 71
for HIV, 35, 71–72, 73–74
for IBS, 96, 97–98, 132 (table)
for MRSA, 66–69, 113
for osteoporosis, 115, 155, 236
for periodontitis, 63, 114, 132
    (table)
for respiratory infections, 69–70,
    118, 148–149
for *S. aureus*, 68
for skin infections, 230
for stomach cancer, 16
for superbugs, 58–60
for tumors, 117

Probiotic products, by illness
    (continued)
    for ulcers, 64–66, 67, 230
    for vaginal infection, 75, 112, 113,
        131, 132 (table)
    for viruses, 69–74
    for yeast infection, 75
Probiotic products, selection of
    age factor for, 125
    allergy factor for, 125
    brands, 126–128, 129
    company reputation in, 121–122
    confusion in, 11, 105–106,
        120–121
    dosage and, 120, 121, 129–131
    drug contraindications in, 124
    label accuracy for, 122, 126–128
    potency factor for, 123
    prebiotic myths and, 107–109
    stability factors for, 122–123
    storage factor for, 125
    vaginal suppositories and, 131
Probiotics
    actions and benefits of, 23–24,
        59–60, 65, 106–107
    for allergies, seasonal, 80, 84–85,
        116, 231
    antibiotics versus, 13–14,
        58–60
    bacteriocins in, 65, 68, 169
    CFUs of, 120, 121, 123
    in cheese, 112, 118
    definition of, 4
    for elderly, 70, 128
    in infants, 117
    killing, 123, 170, 172, 176
    in media, 3
    for pets, 128
    powder, 144

at pregnancy, 84, 101, 110,
        115–116, 124
    shelf life of, 123
    side effects of, 121
    trademarks on, 137–138
    in yogurt, 133–138, 155, 160,
        234–235, 236
    See also Fermented foods
Propionibacterium acnes, P. acnes,
        68
Propionibacterium freudenreichii,
        P. freudenreichii, 68
Prostate cancer, 159
Protease, 43
Protein sources, 39–41, 193
Proteus, 77
Psoriasis, 36
Psychological disorders, 85–86,
        103–105, 231
Pumpkin seed cheese, 203–204

RA. *See* Rheumatoid arthritis
Radiation therapy, 90–91, 238
Recipes
    beverages, 193–198
    cheese, 199–205
    desserts, 216–223
    salad dressings, 205–207
    vegetable ferments, 207–216
    yogurt, 186–192
Red pepper soft cheese, 201–202
Respiratory infections
    fermented foods for, 148–149,
        239–240
    probiotics for, 69–70, 118,
        148–149
Resveratrol, 140
Rheumatoid arthritis (RA), 87–88,
        232

Rhinoconjunctivitis, 84
Roasted Red Pepper Soft Cheese, 201–202
Rotavirus, 116, 117
Russia
    fermented foods from, 148, 175
    research from, 64, 148, 154, 175, 236
Ryhanen, Eeva-Liisa, 238

Saccharomyces boulardii, S. boulardii, 67, 101, 119
Saccharomyces cerevisiae, S. cerevisiae, 80, 85
SAD. See Standard American Diet
St. John's Wort, 104
Salad dressings, 205–207
Saliva, 31–32, 236
Salmonella, 150, 167, 169
Salt
    about, 184–185
    for brining, 144
    for grain or legume fermentation, 146–147
Sauerkraut
    benefits of, 166–169, 238
    fermentation process, 171–172, 238
    origins, 168–169
    recipes, 171, 208–211
    store-bought, 170
Savory Dairy-Free Greek-Style Yogurt, 188–191
Seeds, 40, 45
    pumpkin seed cheese, 203–204
    sunflower seed yogurt, 188–191
Selenium, 102
Sex
    Candida from, 29

gonorrhea, 55–56, 77
herpes, 71
Shelf life, 123, 177
Shigella, 167, 169
Shinya, Hiromi, 14
Shiva, Vandana, 181
Side effects
    of antibiotics, diarrhea, 60–63
    of chemotherapy, 90–91
    of probiotics, 121
Simple Sauerkraut, 208–209
Sinusitis, 79–80, 85
Skin problems
    acne, 50
    aging, 155–156
    antibiotics and, 50, 230
    cancer, 139–141
    dermatitis, 239
    eczema, 36, 84
    fermented foods for, 155–156, 174, 176–177, 239
    wound treatment, 176–177, 239–240
Slovakia, 232–233
Smith, Leonard, 35
Smoking, 91
Smoothies, 193–194
Sodium, 146–147, 164, 239
Soft and Creamy Dairy-Free Cheese, 199–200
Sourdough bread, 147
Soy
    miso, 163–165, 237–238
    myths, 157–160, 164
    nutrient absorption from, 149, 164
    prebiotics and, 156–157
    protein sources, 40
    tofu, 165
    yogurt, 151–157, 186–188, 235, 236

SpA. *See* Spondyloarthritis
Spain, 235
Spondyloarthritis (SpA), 232
Standard American Diet (SAD), 33,
    38, 113
Staphylococcus, 77, 169
Staphylococcus aureus, S. aureus, 55,
    68, 113
Starters, 144–145, 147
Stevia, 43, 185
Stewart, William, 54
Stomach cancer, 15–17
Stool testing, 24
Storage, 125
Strawberries 'N' Cream Smoothie, 194
Streptococcus salivarius
    thermophilus, S. salivarius
    thermophilus, 71, 133
Streptococcus thermophilus,
    S. thermophilus, 132 (table)
    about, 118–119
    antibiotics and, 59, 62
    for diabetes, 92
    for IBS, 97
    in yogurt, 154, 234
Streptomycin, 56, 57, 59
Stress
    Candida from, 29, 48
    digestive problems and, 42, 83,
        85–86
Sugar
    allergies from, 80
    alternatives to, 43, 185–186
    in Beer, 27
    Candida from, 28
    depression from, 103–104
    diabetes and, 92–93
    fermentation and, 171–172,
        185–186

in frozen food, 2
oligosaccharides as good, 108–109,
    156–157
in yogurt, 9, 135–136
Sulfanomides, 57
Sun damage, 139–141
Sunflower seed yogurt, 188–191
Sunlight therapy, 105
Superbugs
    creation of, 54–57
    dandelion for, 76
    probiotics for, 58–60
    rise of, 49–54
Superoxide dismutase, 17
Sweden, 89, 229
Sweet Yogurt, 191–192
Sweeteners, 185–186
    See also Sugar
"Swing voter" bacteria, 19–20
Symptom suppression, 10

Taiwan, 168–169, 237
Tamoxifen, 237
Tea
    herbal, 43, 119
    kombucha, 175–177, 195–198,
        239–240
Teitelbaum, Jacob, 26
Temperature, 227
Testosterone, 233
Tests, diagnostic, 24
Tetanus, 117
Tetracycline, 53, 57, 59
Thyme cheese, 202–203
Tofu, 165
Trademarks, 137–138
Transposons, 53
Traveler's diarrhea, 99, 132 (table)
    See also Food poisoning

Triclosan, 50
Tumors, 117
   See also Cancer
Turkey (country), 147, 161
Turmeric, 17, 140

Ukraine, 71
Ulcerative colitis, 36, 94, 118
Ulcers, 64–66, 67, 198, 230
Urinary tract infections, 55

Vaginal infection
   douches for, 72, 131
   HIV and, 73
   probiotics for, 75, 112, 113, 131,
      132 (table)
   suppositories for, 131
   yeast, 75–78
   See also Candida
Vagus nerve, 86
Vancomycin, 59
Vanilla Coconut Cream, 217
Vanilla Coconut Ice Cream,
   218–219
Vanilla Frozen Yogurt, 221–222
Vegetables
   about, 183–184
   antibiotics used on, 56–57
   cabbage kimchi, 172–175,
      214–216, 238–239
   cabbage sauerkraut, 166–172,
      208–211, 238
   carrots, 211–212
   ferment recipes, 207–216
   freshness preservation of, 141–142,
      179
   green bean pickles, 213
   hot sauce, 212
   onions, 214

Veterinary antibiotics, 51
Villi, intestinal, 32, 33, 83,
   93–94
Vinaigrette, 206–207
Vinegar, 43, 146
Viruses
   AIDS, 72, 73–74
   herpes, 71
   HIV, 35, 71–72, 73–74
   leaky gut and, 36
   natural remedies for, 75–78
   probiotics for, 69–74
   superbugs and, 50, 53
   See also Flu
VitaClay, 183
Vitamins
   for aging, 102
   for chronic fatigue, 49
   definition of, 31
   for depression, 86, 104
   in kefir, 161
   in kombucha, 175

Waste, 179
Water, 28, 131, 162
   intake, 44, 108, 130
Weight gain, 26–27, 237
Weissella, 173
Whey
   about, 186
   Dairy-Free Whey, 188
   Savory Dairy-Free Greek-Style
      Yogurt, 190–191
   starter, 145
Wodskou, Chris, 51
Women, estrogen balance in, 30, 149,
   158–159, 168
   See also Breast cancer; Vaginal
      infection

World Health Organization, 1
Wound treatment, 176–177,
    239–240

Xenoestrogen, 30, 158–159

Yeast
    in alcoholic fermentation, 145
    in kombucha, 240
    S. boulardii, 67, 101, 119
    S. cerevisiae, 80, 85
    in sourdough bread, 147
Yeast infection, 75–78
    See also Candida
Yoga, 46
Yogurt
    almond, 186–192
    benefits of, 74, 148–150, 153–157,
        230–231
    brands, 135–138

cashew, 188–192
dairy-free, 151–157, 186–192,
    234–235, 236
frozen, 221–222
Greek-style, 188–191
history of, 147–148
homemade, 134–135, 157,
    186–188
marketing gimmicks, 136–138
probiotics in, 133–138, 155, 160,
    234–235, 236
problems with, 135–138, 150–151,
    152–153
recipes, 186–192
soy, 151–157, 186–188, 235, 236
starter, 144–145
sugar in, 9, 135–136
sunflower seed, 188–191

Zygosaccharomyces, 240